Patienthood and Communication

Health Communication

Gary L. Kreps, Series Editor

Vol. 13

The Health Communication series is part of
the Peter Lang Media and Communication list.
Every volume is peer reviewed and meets
the highest quality standards for content and production.

PETER LANG
New York • Bern • Frankfurt • Berlin
Brussels • Vienna • Oxford • Warsaw

Peter M. Kellett

Patienthood and Communication

A Personal Narrative of Eye Disease and Vision Loss

PETER LANG
New York • Bern • Frankfurt • Berlin
Brussels • Vienna • Oxford • Warsaw

Library of Congress Cataloging-in-Publication Data

Names: Kellett, Peter M., author.
Title: Patienthood and communication: a personal narrative of
eye disease and vision loss / Peter M. Kellett.
Description: New York: Peter Lang, 2017.
Series: Health communication; vol. 13 | ISSN 2153-1277
Includes bibliographical references and index.
Identifiers: LCCN 2017020653 | ISBN 9781433138300 (paperback: alk. paper)
ISBN 978-1-4331-3831-7 (hardback: alk. paper)
ISBN 978-1-4331-4574-2 (ebook PDF)
ISBN 978-1-4331-4575-9 (epub) | ISBN 978-1-4331-4576-6 (mobi)
Subjects: LCSH: Kellett, Peter M.,—Health. | Retinal
degeneration—Patients—Biography. | Eye—Diseases—
Patients—Biography.
Communication in medicine. | Communication in families.
Classification: LCC RE661.D3 K45 2017 | DDC 362.1977/350092 [B]—dc23
LC record available at https://lccn.loc.gov/2017020653
DOI 10.3726/b12052

Bibliographic information published by **Die Deutsche Nationalbibliothek**.
Die Deutsche Nationalbibliothek lists this publication in the "Deutsche
Nationalbibliografie"; detailed bibliographic data are available
on the Internet at http://dnb.d-nb.de/.

29 Broadway, 18th floor, New York, NY 10006
www.peterlang.com

CONTENTS

ACKNOWLEDGEMENTS

I would like to thank my wife, Hema, for always being there as we lived through the first five years of this story together. I truly appreciate all of her coaching, and supportive and caring communication that held me together as I went through this experience. Thanks to my mother and father, Mary and Albert Kellett, and David, Tim and Paul, my brothers—they have all helped me in their own unique and personal ways. In particular I acknowledge David, my twin brother, who also shares this disease—we are bound together by our genes for the good, the bad, and the ugly! Thanks also to my Indian Family: Dad, Mummy-Ji, Chitti and Jayanth, Reena, Deepak, and Sagarika. The relational communication and friendship of several friends have been crucial in keeping me positive and hopeful in this journey. These include: John Gribble, Art Murphy, Steve Kroll-Smith, John Nostrand, Alie Buckley, Bud Goodall (deceased), Joe Gemin, and others.

I owe much gratitude to my care-full Medical and professional team. These include: Dr. Johnson of Oman Eye Care. Dr. Jason Sanders of Piedmont Retina Specialists, Dr. Vishak John of Wake Forest Baptist Medical Center, and Dr. Phil Rosenfeld and Cristy Lage-Rodriguez at Bascom-Palmer Eye Institute at the University of Miami. Thank you all for helping me so much. Thanks also to the hard working, dedicated, accessible, and kind people at the Lowy Medical Research Institute (LMRI), particularly Jennifer Trombley, Dr. Lea Scheppke, and Dr. Martin Friedlander. Keep up the great work!

Special thanks goes the Lowy family for their vision and generosity in funding the research into MacTel. We are on the verge of unlocking its mystery, and all the good that this will bring, because of you.

I would also like to thank all of my colleagues and friends in the Disability Issues Caucus of the National Communication Association for enabling me to develop and present my ideas relevant to this book at the conference.

Finally, I would like to add a personal note of thanks to series editor Gary Kreps for his encouragement and the freedom he has allowed me to tell this story just as I lived it.

INTRODUCTION

Health Communication—An Eye-Patient's View

Immediately after being diagnosed with degenerative retinal disease in 2011, I began journaling the experience. I had never been a journal keeper, but something compelled me to document the fine fabric of this unfolding story in which I suddenly and unexpectedly found myself. I wrote what I thought were the important moments along the way. I tried to remember important and interesting conversations as they were happening, and write them down as soon as I could. I tried to capture the internal (thoughts and feelings) and external (talk and behavior) aspects of my experiences, and the context of the time and place physically and relationally that they occurred, as I knew these details would soon disappear from memory with time. What follows is a synthesis of these journal notes into the story—my personal narrative account—of the first five years of adapting to a disease (MacTel) that would cause me progressive and irreversible vision-loss. The story is told in short chapters that are most often organized around, and punctuated by, diagnostic and treatment moments in order to capture the centrality of the disease and treatment to these five years. At the same time, experiential and relational themes recur, interweave, and change/evolve across the span of the five years, and each chapter reflects this interweaving of thematic threads.

Oddly, in retrospect, although I was engrossed with documenting my experience, journaling it allowed me a slight externalizing distance from it that was helpful and healthy. At times, I felt like I was just writing an interesting story in which I happened to be a character. Although, looking back, there were times when I did not always like how my character talked, thought, and behaved, it was distance that helped me to cope with the fear of uncertainty and looming blindness, and all that emanated from that fear. At the same time, in confronting the flaws of my own character—my propensity at times in the story to dwell in denial and fear; my slowness to take charge of the treatment; my patterns of responses that were often suffused with anger, disappointment, and self-pity, there was the opportunity for important learning and growth as a patient. For me, the meaning of patienthood was transformed as I embraced learning and growth as part of the disease process, and when I empowered myself to more actively and skillfully author the events that I now story here.

Crucially, the experience of these early stages of retinal disease and related vision loss taught me a great deal about the constant interweaving of communication and the disease experience in the lived experience of everyday life. The ongoing dynamics of relational and health care communication, and my particular disease experience, provide valuable insights and lessons more generally for those interested in health communication. Here, I will briefly explore the insights into the relationship between communication and disease I experienced through each of the five years documented, and where possible connect such insights to health communication more broadly.

The first seven chapters constitute part one of the book, and represent my experience of the first year with eye disease and vision loss. Part one tells the story of the first year (2011–2012), from diagnosis through early treatment. The year began with a regular check-up at the optometrist office. My optometrist noticed dark rings around my retinas and insisted that I go to an ophthalmologist. Suddenly I was a patient. More shocking, I was diagnosed with a degenerative disease for which there is currently no treatment or known cure. I sought information, definition, clarity, but there was little help I could find either in person from health care providers, or online. My early attempts to make sense and adjust through adaptation and communication in a low information quality environment are documented (Johnson & Case, 2012), as are the impacts of this shock on my sense of self, and my close personal relationships and priorities (Miller-Day, 2011).

In November 2011, I experienced dizziness and visual distortion but was put off from going back to my ophthalmologist until December at the six month mark, as planned. On returning to my ophthalmologist on December 23rd I was told that my right retina was swelling and bleeding, and that I needed an Avastin injection immediately. Poignantly, I was the last patient there, holding up their office Christmas party.

I describe the four monthly injections to follow that year, and the emotional, relational, and communicative impact of this intense period of treatment to save my right eye, which thankfully worked. Particularly noted are the impacts on, and impacts of, close personal, and familial relationships (Miller-Day, 2011).

As the first year closed, I also reflect on the various and often competing "voices" I was hearing on how I ought to understand and relate to this disease. The medical discourse was telling me one thing. Friends and family members were telling me other things. Sometimes these voices were competing, and they were often confusing. I had to learn how to sift through what people were telling me for ways forward *for myself*. I also had to learn how to tell people about the disease, and to not misunderstand their reactions and responses. I had to live without clarity, both of my vision and of relevant information. Finally, I also had to learn how to better balance the often competitive struggle between the dark and the bright side—between fear, anger, disappointment, and despair on the one hand, and hope, gratitude, and optimism on the other (Pitts & Socha, 2013; Socha & Pitts, 2012).

Chapter's eight through eleven document my experience of the second year with the disease, represented as part two of the book. The second year began with the sixth injection into my right eye. It had responded well to treatment, and I was asked to return in eight weeks instead of six for the next injection. That stretch of two weeks was good news, a victory even. After this injection, and after spending some considerable time in waiting rooms and doctor's offices, I reflect on the communication I experienced in these contexts. I also describe the rituals my wife, Hema, and I instituted to celebrate completing each treatment. I characterize this period as a "muddling through." I had to adapt and change how I read. I tried to adapt to difficulty recognizing faces, and many other everyday communicative activities. For example, I became clumsier because of blind spots which, at different times, was a source or both relational frustration, stress, and humor for Hema and me (Hamilton & Vecksler, 2014; Scholl, 2013; Wanzer, Booth-Butterfield, & Booth-Butterfield, 2005).

I rekindled my long-time friendship with Bud Goodall, and our common health care experiences—his with terminal pancreatic cancer and mine with my disease, sparked a fascinating online back and forth of support, celebration, and humor, which continued until his death (Kellett, 2012, 2013; Meyer, 2000, 2012; Scholl, 2013).

Hema and I travelled to England and India to meet each other's families, then I returned for my seventh injection which was my last, for now. I was declared a "success story" although I still had no definitive idea what disease I actually had, or why I had it. This began to pull at me as an uncomfortable mystery that needed addressing. I returned to school after a year away on research leave. My pal, Bud Goodall, died. My twin brother began tests for eye problems he was having, and a parallel if different journey as twins, across two continents and two health care systems, began to take shape.

During the rest of this year I document awkward moments, scary moments, dangerous moments, humorous moments, and poignant moments. Along with these, there were meaningful moments of connection with other people with similar eye problems, which I craved by this point in my journey.

Chapter's twelve and thirteen tell the story of the third year of my disease and vision loss journey. Part three of this book begins with Hema's parents visiting us from India to be part of our wedding. As we all get to know each other at close quarters, they begin to understand the everyday dynamics of my vision issues and how they affected Hema and mine's everyday relationship.

I wrote and published my first paper on ocular health and disease and its impact on communication (Kellett, 2014). So began a major shift in my scholarly interests and identity around eye health, vision loss, and disability (Kellett, Buckley, & Frame, 2016; Kellett, 2017).

I travelled to Budapest alone to present a paper at a conference, and found the experience challenging and difficult. I also realized how much I had come to rely on Hema, and how fearful I had become when outside my comfort zone. In a classic dialectical tension, this reliance on the familiar was a source of frustration for her, but desired safety for me.

After the wedding, we went on honeymoon together after Hema's parent left, and several humorous vision related moments are described.

Upon returning to school, I was teaching a graduate class in "Positive Communication" for the first time. In my introduction on day one, I told the class how my experiences with communication during my vision loss had been instrumental in my interest in creating and teaching this class. Simply, I told them that what people said to me along the way had saved me from despair and given me hope and comfort, and I wanted to explore this aspect of communication in a scholarly as well as personally meaningful way (Sullivan, 2013).

A few of my close friends began to share health challenges, and we began to weave our health related narratives together, in amongst other things we shared. Whether good news at the Cardiologist, or with a prostate condition, or with my eyes, support and celebration of good news—stability (however fleeting and even perhaps mythical)—was enormously helpful for each of us (Bodie & Burleson, 2008; Burleson, 2003, 2010; Burleson & MacGeorge, 2002; McCullough & Burleson, 2012).

My eye acuity returned to a much better 20/70 as the retinal swelling reduced more, and I put vision issues out of my mind as much as possible—enjoying the stability. There were moments, however, that reminded me of how fragile the myth and reality of "stability" were when set against its dialectical partner —decline—in a degenerative disease path.

The fourth year (Part four) is captured by chapter's fourteen through seventeen. The fourth year began with a return to the Piedmont Retina Clinic for a one year check-up. Although the news was good—no swelling, and my edemas were dry, my retinas had thinned and I had many other unanswered questions. I did not believe I had Cone-Dystrophy, but I did not really know what disease I did have. I announced that I had decided to seek further advice at a "research" hospital, and this essentially ended my relationship with my ophthalmologist up until that point. It did, however, begin for me a much more proactive and empowered approach to my health care (Ledford, Caffrey, & Russell, 2015). I sought a second opinion at Wake Forest Baptist Medical Center and was diagnosed as having MacTel. I had previously been misdiagnosed. My Twin brother, David, was also going through a similar diagnostic process in London. He was eventually diagnosed with the same condition, indicating a genetic origin of the disease for both of us. We began to share experiences online in the form of short comments back and forth on Facebook Messenger. I joined the MacTel Project Group on Facebook. David and I began the long process of donating our genes to the MacTel Project's global genetic study that was already underway.

My North Carolina driver's license was due for renewal on my upcoming birthday, causing me much stress and worry about independence, and related issues, although I probably would have passed the vision test given how much my eyes had stabilized. My brother's license was revoked in England, causing him more stress and worry than I had, as I was able to renew mine online.

Hema and I went to Bascom-Palmer Eye Center in Miami so that I could be officially diagnosed with MacTel by one of the MacTel Project ophthalmologists, and to donate a genetic sample for the research study. I also signed forms to donate my eyes to the clinic upon my death. David did not get to donate his genes for a while longer as they were, by this point, prioritizing the search for other family members with MacTel rather than direct siblings. Hema landed her dream job (or so she thought at the time), which meant she would not be available to help me as much on things I struggled with, but which also meant that she would be able to take care of herself irrespective of what happened to me. The ability to be independent was my dream for her, as much as it was my dream for myself, albeit in a different way.

Finally, the fifth year (Part five) of this experience is narrated through chapter's eighteen through twenty one. Year five began with some reflection on the typical miscommunications that occur because of my low-vision condition. I began to be more proactive in dealing with such miscommunications. I also shared information about my eye condition more openly with students, some of whom surprised me by sharing information about their own eye and vision issues. In some cases this mutual disclosure became a sources of deeper connection between us.

I returned to Wake Forest for a check-up and, ominously, "two small red dots" on my left retina ushered in a period of more close observation and related worry. I was invited to give a talk to their residents and fellows which I agreed to do in the summer. I was also invited by the LMRI to share my story as a patient with MacTel to be featured on their website as part of their new informational and communication initiative (LMRI.net).

Hema and I revisited the topic of us having a child. We agreed to put fears of my possible future blindness, and the potential risk of passing the disease on to any child we might have, aside and try to start a family.

Vision loss, health, and disability became a closer part of my professional and personal identity. I got involved with the Disability Issues Caucus of the National Communication Association, and began talks with other faculty on my campus to create an academic program in Disability Studies.

Everyday struggles with vision and its interconnections with relationships, particularly around support and humor, are explored and exemplified.

I returned to Wake Forest for a check-up, and all seemed stable again. The red dots had disappeared for now—just as mysteriously as they had appeared. As Dr. John and I became closer and better acquainted, I firmed up plans with him to come and give a talk, and possibly to be part of their design process—providing them with a patient's perspective on interior design for their new building which was, as yet, at the "dream stage."

I pushed myself to become more productive with the writing and editing of several books I had planned (including this one), and I resolved to get these done before further vision decline occurred, which would make these things much more difficult.

My story was the first to be featured on the LMRI website, and this opened up more online and social media based involvement and connection for me with other patients (Yang, 2017). More people agreed to share their stories for use on the LMRI website. I shared the link to the interview with many people, and this also opened up communication in some interesting and meaningful ways.

Part five ends with a poignant domestic scene of supportive cooperation and complementarity of strengths. As Hema spotted the first of the ripe figs at the tops of our fig bushes—something I would find difficult—I pulled down the heavy branches for us to pick them together—something she would find difficult—and so, with this organic metaphor, the story of our relationship with this disease continued through that summer and on into year six.

References

Bodie, G. D., & Burleson, B. R. (2008). Explaining variations in the effects of supportive messages: A dual process framework. *Communication Yearbook*, *32*, 354–398.

Burleson, B. R. (2003). Emotional support skills. In J. O. Greene & B. R. Burleson (Eds.), *Handbook of communication and social interaction skills* (pp. 551–594). Mahwah, NJ: Erlbaum.

Burleson, B. R. (2010). Explaining recipient responses to supportive messages: Development and tests of a dual-process theory. In S. W. Smith & S. R. Wilson (Eds.), *New directions in interpersonal communication* (pp. 159–179). Thousand Oaks, CA: Sage.

Burleson, B. R., & MacGeorge, E. L. (2002). Supportive communication. In M. L. Knapp & J. A. Daly (Eds.), *Handbook of interpersonal communication* (3rd ed., pp. 374–424). Thousand Oaks, CA: Sage.

Hamilton, M. A., & Vecksler, A. E. (2014). Types of stress and their effect on mental health, verbal aggression, and assault. In J. A. Honeycutt, C. R. Sawyer, & S. A. Keaton (Eds.), *The influence of communication on physiology and health*. (pp. 153–170). New York, NY and Bern, Switzerland: Peter Lang.

Johnson, J. D., & Case, D. O. (2012). *Health information seeking*. New York, NY and Bern, Switzerland: Peter Lang.

Kellett, P. M. (2012). Intersecting narratives—Positive communication. In A. de la Garza, R. L. Krizek, & N. Trujillo (Eds.), *Celebrating bud: A Festschrift in honor of the life & work of H.L. "Bud" Goodall, Jr.* (pp. 121–125). Arizona State University, Inquiry Press.

Kellett, P. M. (2013, Winter). Mutually supportive communication and relational narratives: Online conversations between two friends in declining health. *Qualitative Communication Research*, *2*(4), 337–355.

Kellett, P. M. (2014). Toward a framework for the study of ocular health and disease: Lessons from a personal narrative of vision loss. In M. Eaves (Ed.), *Applications in health communication: Emerging trends* (pp. 217–230). Dubuque, IA: Kendall-Hunt.

Kellett, P. M. (2017). Disability and communication. In M. Allen (Ed.), *The SAGE Encyclopedia of communication research methods*. Thousand Oaks, CA: Sage.

Kellett, P. M., Buckley, A. N., & Frame, M. J. (2016). Communication, teaching and learning, and faculty disability: Lessons from a personal narrative. In A. Atay & M. Z. Ashlock (Eds.), *The discourse of disability in communication education: Narrative-based research for social change* (pp. 11–27). New York, NY: Peter Lang.

Ledford, C. J. W., Caffrey, L. A., & Russell, T. C. (2015). The influence of health literacy on patient information seeking and change. *Journal of Health Communication, 20*, 77–82.

Meyer, J. C. (2000). Humor as a double-edged sword: Four functions of humor in communication. *Communication Theory, 10(3)*, 310–331.

Meyer, J. C. (2012). Humor as personal relationship enhances: Positivity for the long term. In T. J. Socha & M. J. Pitts (Eds.), *The positive side of interpersonal communication* (pp. 161–178). New York, NY: Peter Lang.

Miller-Day, M. (2011). *Family communication, connections, and health transitions: Going through this together*. New York, NY and Bern, Switzerland: Peter Lang.

Pitts, M. J., & Socha, T. J. (Eds.). (2013). *Positive communication in health and wellness*. New York, NY and Bern, Switzerland: Peter Lang.

Scholl, J. C. (2013). Humor as a tool, not a therapy: A preliminary model of humor in health communication. In M. J. Pitts & T. J. Socha (Eds.), *Positive communication in health and wellness* (pp. 43–62). New York, NY: Peter Lang.

Socha, T. J., & Pitts, M. J. (Eds.). (2012). *The positive side of interpersonal communication*. New York, NY and Bern, Switzerland: Peter Lang.

Sullivan, C. F. (2013). Positive relational communication: Impact on health. In M. J. Pitts & T. J. Socha (Eds.), *Positive communication in health and wellness* (pp. 29–42). New York, NY: Peter Lang.

Wanzer, M., Booth-Butterfield, M., & Booth-Butterfield, S. (2005). "If we didn't use humor, we'd cry": Humorous coping communication in health care settings. *Journal of Health Communication, 10*(2), 105–125.

Yang, Q. (2017). Are social media sites making health behavior change interventions more effective? A meta-analytic review. *Journal of Health Communication, 22*, 223-233.

YEAR 1

Mid-May 2011 to Mid-May 2012

· 1 ·

A DOUBLE BULLS-EYE

"Have you ever been a sun-gazer?"

It was a bright, sunny, afternoon in mid-May, 2011 when I finally got around to getting my eyes checked for the first time in at least two years. I had switched to a new optometrist who had been recommended to me by several people. I breezed in, ready to get the updated prescription I needed in order to get new glasses, most likely at the adjoining glasses shop. I had noticed for some time that my old prescription was out of date. Squinting over them to do emails, struggling to read the small print of books and magazines, difficulty seeing at night, and other small clues had built up and nagged at me to get an appointment. I do not know why I always seemed to put off eye exams until it was obvious my prescription was out of date but, like many others, I did. My old glasses were also just simply "done." One of the arms had started to come off regularly leaving me trying to replace the tiny screw to fix them. The screws in the repair kits I picked up at Walgreen's never quite worked perfectly and, even if they did, it was nearly impossible to do the repair without actually wearing my glasses.

The arm of my glasses had slipped off most recently right before my very last faculty meetings as department head. I did not have the repair kit with me at the office so I had to go into the meeting with broken glasses—one arm missing. I apologized playfully up front, hoping to head off any comments before people noticed. There were some giggles, and a couple of snide comments to the effects that this was symbolic of the coming end of my term as head. The glasses were done, and so was I! I was embarrassed that they had the opportunity to make this joke at my expense, but it was an obvious one to make, and I could not blame them for grabbing the low hanging fruit. It was partly true and, anyway, why not begin another dull meeting with a laugh?

I was ready for new glasses—updated in prescription, stylish, and that would be ready for the summer when I would be going to England on vacation, and that would see me into the research leave coming in August and beyond. It was a good time to change them, I had free time after getting through the last hurrah of the departmental graduation celebration (hoping nervously that my glasses would not break on stage while I hosted the event), and all of the paper work that leads up to it. I had unburdened myself of a huge amount of paper and clutter as I cleared out my office, and filled the large "confidential recycling bin" in the department. Life was lighter all round, and the afternoon was similarly bright and full of hope. A friend had planned to join me after the eye test to help me pick out new frames, and I was looking forward to that.

"I have never seen anything like this" the optometrist stated as she came back into the testing room.

"What do you mean?" I asked, feeling almost an accusatory tone in her voice as well as the shock of this unexpected turn in the script.

"You have these shadowy areas around the optic nerves at the back of your eyes," she replied.

"Oh yes?" I inquired, looking at the black and white images she was showing me, and growing more concerned. The usual script of "here is your prescription, see you next time" that we had strayed from was being replaced with a new, unexpected one for both of us. She seemed as thrown off her routine as I was.

"What is that?" I asked, hoping it was not much to worry about beyond a normal sign of aging.

"Well, we're going to have to send you to a retina specialist to figure out what's going on with your retinas" she responded. "But we're seeing what's known as a bulls-eye pattern here. And you're a young man, you shouldn't have this!"

Again, I felt a little accused, although I was sure I was just in mild shock at the surreal conversation we both found ourselves in. What had I done wrong to have this bulls-eye pattern, and what did it mean? I was fumbling around in my head for clues, but none came to me. Probably like most people, I knew almost nothing about retinas at that point in my life, beyond the usual analogy of them being like the film in an old-fashioned camera. I had no family or immediate friends with such problems that I knew of, and so, I had no exposure to retinal diseases. I had always just gone to the optometrist every year or two, had the dreary letter tests and gotten new glasses based on the normal changes they found. This was an abrupt and shocking departure.

"Have you ever been a sun-gazer?" She asked.

"What's that?" I responded.

"Someone who gazes at the sun", she said seriously and without even the slightest irony.

"No" I responded, thinking to myself what the hell kind of a question is this—"a sun-gazer"? What is she saying here, I wondered? I was starting to get flustered.

"Is there a link to sunlight or sun damage for whatever this is"? I asked, regrouping to ask what I thought might be a smart question, given her line of thought.

"I don't know," she said "but this is something we see usually in elderly people. You're only (she glanced at my papers) 48 and shouldn't have this."

Later, I realized that her shock was understandable, and that she was not being accusatory at all. I was just feeling defensive at the strange and disturbing news unfolding. I read somewhere online later that day that this bulls-eye pattern affects only one in 30,000 people when it is not age related. So, I assumed that in her practice she had probably never come across this before. There were, maybe, a couple of other people in Greensboro with this condition, if the statistics held true. After all these years thinking myself lucky to dodge whatever came around and affected people I know, I was suddenly a statistic—a "case of …" something I did not even have a name for yet, but which looked like a bulls-eye target around each optic nerve. But, was there a better question to lead off with than, "Have you ever been a sun-gazer?!" I did not even know what that was, and it only added to the confusion and strangeness of the moment.

I was stunned when she went on to tell me that they would not give me a prescription to get new glasses until they had been cleared to do so by a retina specialist. I would not get new glasses until they were convinced that it was worth it for me to buy new ones. I gulped and swallowed uncomfortably and felt my body reacting in all kinds of ways that felt like alarm, fight—flight, and shock. "WHAT" … I thought to myself … "IT MIGHT NOT BE *WORTH IT?*" Hearing this was a really heavy moment. It took away my last opportunity for momentary denial. The last part of the script I expected to play out when I walked in had been ripped away and all I had left was what she was directing me to do next. Could they not have gone ahead and let me have an updated prescription anyway as if things were ok? They were right to handle it this way but, at the time, I did not know what else to think.

The rest of that afternoon is a blur, but I do remember calling my friend and telling her not to come. I would not be picking out new glasses until I saw a specialist, and maybe not even then if the news was as bad as perhaps it could be. I also remember the people at the optometrist office setting up the appointment with the retina specialist for me, which was kind. My optometrist was also keen to assure me that the retina specialist was brilliant, as well as a really nice young local guy who had come back to his home town to set up his specialty practice. They said that retina specialists are not always nice to them as Optometrists, but that he was always nice. This was another of many odd statements that I did not understand at the time. I was unfamiliar with the relational world of optometrists and ophthalmologists (which I also found to be a very strange word at first). Anyway, I had an appointment to meet with Dr. Sanders just a week or two later. I was in enough shock that I cannot recall many of my thoughts or conversations from the rest of that day.

Taking stock as a way to manage the stress of the moment, I told myself I could still see fairly well. The morning and evenings were lighter now in the springtime which made driving relatively easy. Night driving had been difficult for me for years already, especially if it was raining. I reassured myself that I had an easy going last few months as department head between now and July 31st, and much to look forward to, so I more or less put it all out of my mind until the appointment with Dr. Sanders crept inevitably around.

A Diagnosis and a Name

A good friend, Hema, took me for my first appointment at Dr. Sanders's office. I paid the co-pay and waited with her. After a short wait, my name was called and I followed the technician into a small square windowless room. I had a letter recognition test and my eyes were then dilated. The drops were uncomfortable but, as the sign in the waiting room stated, dilation was necessary for all visits to a retina specialist. I noticed the sign and wondered if patients had tried to refuse the dilation, or habitually complained about it. Oddly, it read like a conversation with an imaginary patient who was questioning the need for the dilation. Perhaps the receptionists just got tired of people asking the same questions about dilation being necessary. I went through a series of tests after my eyes had been dilated. The technician broke the silence in the image/picture taking room.

"You remind me of someone famous. I am trying to think of his name," she said.

"Really"? I asked, hoping for the best. After all she was an expert with images!

"Pauly Shore" She said, after thinking for a moment.

"Really"? I said. "I haven't ever heard that one."

"I Like Pauly Shore" she said, "he's funny"—I think clarifying slightly so I took it as a compliment.

"Where are you from?" she went on to ask. We chatted a little about where we were both from. I think she was helping to making me feel comfortable, which definitely helped. After all, this was a surreal and bizarre moment in which to find myself—being tested for retinal disease. The lightness of the chatter definitely helped offset the heaviness of the moment.

The technician injected a dye substance into my bloodstream and then, after a minute, she took pictures of my retinas with bright flashes of light that made the room appear one color then another—red then green. I looked up and right, down and left, down and right then up and left, and straight ahead. Several pictures were taken of each eye pose. Finally they were done. The images were saved and forwarded to the doctor, and I was on to the next examining room, where I was led to wait for Dr. Sanders. While waiting, I wondered momentarily about how all of this would have been done just a few years ago, before all of this high tech digital imaging and computer technology surrounding me. What would such a visit have been like even just 20 years ago? No one here had the length of experience to know first-hand. The diagnostic technology now was impressive. I sat there hoping that the treatment side of the process would also be as advanced as the diagnostics. I relaxed a little, and waited for the doctor. I had a trusty but decidedly low tech pad and pen ready at my side with which to take notes on whatever he was about to tell me.

After perhaps ten minutes I finally met Dr. Sanders. He was young, smart, and I could tell he was a caring soul right from the start. Oddly he had been a student at Clemson University while I had taught there as a brand new assistant professor fresh out of grad school many years ago. He did not have me as a professor, which would have been a really interesting twist in the story, but we shared a brief conversation about the place back then. I remembered the terrible dorm he said he lived in, which was notorious for having metal walls—a throwback to the days when dorms were basic quarters for the cadets. It had since been demolished and replaced right before I left with a nice new modern set of Apartment suites designed, as they were these days, to help attract and retain new students. Our paths would cross more directly here almost 20 years later as doctor and patient. Here we were at Piedmont Retina in Greensboro, North Carolina. I could never have imagined.

Even stranger than our contemporaneous history at Clemson, he asked me the same question my optometrist asked, the one about whether or not I had ever been a sun-gazer. Perhaps this really is the first diagnostic question for this type of condition. Just as I did before, I asked him what he meant. He clarified by saying some people like to take psychotropic drugs and stare at the sun. Psychotropic drugs? Was I being profiled based on my profession and longer hair, I wondered? I assured him I had never been a sun-gazer, although in the back of my mind I wondered if being out in the sun, especially sun bathing with or without sunglasses, might also be connected to the shadowy pattern my optometrist had first noticed. Could this be sun damage? As bizarre sounding as sun-gazing was, sun bathing and being out in the sun without eye protection was much more commonplace, and certainly something I had done regularly in the summer time over the years. What if I had unknowingly done this to myself by not knowing to better protect my eyes? He went on to ask if I had a family history of this or other eye conditions. I could not think of anyone in the family who had eye trouble. My parents did not even wear glasses, and they were in their late 70's at the time. Perhaps this was just a good place to start—one genetic oriented question and one environmental—but the questioning just sort of ended there. Perhaps the rest was a mystery for him too at this point. I did not understand the thinking behind the questions.

He went on to tell me that he had diagnosed the pattern on my retinas as "Bulls-eye Cone Dystrophy" a degenerative disease of the macula part of the retina. He went on to explain that this is a type of maculopathy normally associated with age but, mirroring my optometrist, he said that in my case this was not age related. Hence, the seemingly odd question about sun-gazing. Perhaps they see this as a possible cause—somewhere to begin examining me for leads. But really, that is the first thought—psychotropic drugs and gazing at the sun?!

Finally I had a name for the condition, which was helpful. I wrote the name of the condition on my pad and committed in my mind to do further research online. He went on immediately to tell me that there was no known cause for the disease, and no known treatment. I was stunned. They did not know what caused it, and there was no known treatment. These were among the three most powerful and heavy words I had heard in my life so far: *NO KNOWN TREATMENT*. WOW! I said these three words to myself in my head a few times. How could he be so definite that there was no knowledge of the cause, and no known cure? How could any and all possibilities simply be closed off with these few words? Was this true and absolute, or simply the extent of what is known at this time, given the limited amount of research on this condition? Perhaps he did not want to give me false hope? Was he aware of any ongoing research out there? In the days to come, many such unanswered questions would bubble out from under, and in reaction to, these defining words and the fear and stress they caused. For now, I was mostly struck by the apparent disconnect—even slight irony—between the diagnostic prowess I had seen and experienced that day, and the statement at the end that there's nothing we can do. Such a disconnection was baffling to me—microscopic documentation and clarity on one end, followed by a vast vagueness that just sort of hung over me.

He went on to tell me that the good news was that I had probably had this for many years, maybe even my whole life, and that there was a chance that it could stabilize or at least be very, very slow in its progression. I had no idea what a slow progression would mean. He said there is probably a genetic component to the disease which made my mind turn naturally to my family. I mentioned that I was a twin and asked whether my brother should get tested. He said that it would probably be a good idea, so I made a mental note to tell him. We would revisit this condition six months from now and, from the tests done today, we would have a starting point of comparison by which he could assert more definitely how my disease was likely to track from here. This sounded reasonable and rational, and even hinted at a promise of more clarity. At this point Dr. Sanders was not unduly alarmed, even though it sounded serious. He thought that I had the disease probably for years and that we would simply keep an eye on it over time. I think he wanted the happy version of the story to be true almost as much as I did.

It felt good to be at least on an observational program and to be in good and caring hands, but would I call this "treatment" when there's apparently no hope of improvement or cure? The bad news—good news format of his talk left me hopeful yet balancing this hope with the terrible fear of the unknown that I would have six months to ponder. I loved good news—bad news jokes, but his organizing the diagnosis into the bad news followed by the good news worked much better for a medical diagnosis. Either way you tell the story it is not pretty, or funny, but I think his way worked better.

I made an appointment with the staff at the front desk for mid-December and walked out with Hema who assured me, repeatedly, that I would be fine as I told her the name of the disease with which I had just been diagnosed. These were the very first of many supportive words across the years that she would give me. I was choking back tears as I said the name out loud, and briefly explained what it meant. I do not remember anything from the rest of that day.

· 2 ·

SIX MONTHS TO REBALANCE

With six months to push this news out of my mind as much as I could, and going into the summer of 2011, I was in positive spirits. I had completed 8 years as department head, and was ready for a complete change. It was going to be a fun summer of travel, enjoying the seasonal weather, gardening, and whatever else happened, with a full year of research leave at the end of it, starting in August. Besides this, I had always thought of myself as a guy who was fortunate—maybe more fortunate than the guy next to me most of the time. Perhaps we all think this way until something reminds us of our fragility and our mortality. Life had always seemed to work out one way or another for me. I had very few if any regrets I could name. I was happy where I was in my life. I was in my late 40's and had never had anything serious wrong with me. I had never spent a night in hospital. Whereas, my twin brother had had two bouts with life threatening cancer, I had never really had anything to worry about. I had never had a prescription in the 25 years while living in the US. I was not the type of person who ran to the doctor every time I had a sniffle or an ache. I had a childhood of "not bothering the doctor" (as my mother would say) unless absolutely necessary. As an adult, I lived a life of healthy exercise which had conditioned me to not seek out diagnoses and medications all the time as many of my American friends seemed to. Rather, I expected things to work their way out naturally most of the time. I still believe that the odds are that this will be true but, of course, the down side to this mentality is that if you rarely get physicals or have things that might need looking at looked at, then it is easy to live in a level of denial about health issues. It is possible to convince yourself that diseases do not happen to you, and then something big might just creep up on your "blind spot" and go untreated.

I never thought I would end up with a disease that might leave me with low vision or even blindness at some, as yet, undefined point in time. Months later, when I talked more about it with my family, I was shocked when my dad said that I had always had "bad eyes"—for him this condition was not surprising as it fit a lifelong pattern he saw in me. But I never thought of myself as having bad eyes, as he thought I did. An obvious thing to him was a complete shock to me. At this point in the treatment process, the reality of that word—blind—had not really sunk in. No one was using the word yet. The symptoms were mild enough that I did not even tell my family until much closer to my second appointment with Dr. Sanders in December.

Searching for Clues

I began to search for information and research data relating to the Bulls-Eye Cone Dystrophy with which I had been diagnosed. Mirroring my doctor's words, I quickly re-encountered the definitive statements that this was a disease of unknown origin and was without a cure. There did not even seem to be that much ongoing research out there on this—at least that I could find. My friend, Alksander, suggested one day, as we were browsing around the Weatherspoon art gallery, that this lack of research was "a numbers game" in that few enough people suffered from this particular disease that research just was not feasible. We were enjoying an exhibit that had to do with identity, and I remember telling him about the recent diagnosis and my desire to see art regularly, not knowing when it would be difficult to do so. I think this was the first mindful adaptation to the condition I made—to make a point of seeing art regularly, which I did.

I did find some studies that suggested a diet rich in antioxidants could have an impact on progression. I resolved to switch even more to a diet based on the fruits and vegetables listed typically as antioxidant rich. That summer I did focus on eating antioxidant rich foods. I also became adept at making smoothies from fruits on the list—including the abundant figs that grew in my yard. 2011 was a long hot dry summer but they seemed to thrive well. The question occurred to me, did consuming foods not rich in antioxidants, or rich in other toxins that undermine the action of antioxidant foods, contribute to decline? I could not find anything online on this aspect of nutrition.

I also found some research that suggested a successful link between the use of stem cell implants and stabilization, or perhaps even reversal, of the disease. It made sense that regeneration of retinal cells would have a positive effect on vision. But as the study dryly pointed out, stem cell treatment was expensive, largely experimental, and not typically covered by insurance. When would such treatment be available to someone like me? Were we close? Everything seemed to be five years away from being where it ought to be. What was keeping this treatment from everyday availability? These were questions that I wanted to know more about, but finding any definitive information was frustratingly elusive.

Occasionally my mind turned to the deeper, darker, irony that we had the technology and investment to be able to blow up our enemies so many times over if we wanted to. At this time in 2011, we were engaged in several hugely expensive wars concurrently throughout the world designed at least in part, to maintain our global interests, and yet we had no idea how to treat what seemed like a simple eye disease. The yardsticks we used to measure greatness were discouraging to say the least. The party line on the disease from all sources I found seemed to be consistent—we had no understanding of the cause, and no cure for this form of maculopathy. Frustratingly, it seemed that there were so many unanswered questions and so few places to turn for informative help. I dreamt of having someone knowledgeable to explain it all to me—an advocate, a coach—but who this would be, I had no idea.

In matters of health, things tend to change quickly for the worse, and slowly for the better. When they change for the worse, the experience can be disruptive, traumatic, shocking, and off-balancing. If our everyday lives, and particularly our relationships, can be characterized partly as consisting of the constructions and co-constructions of particular dialectical tensions held in balance for us as normalcy, then quick change can throw us into the struggle to rebalance. Such a struggle can have us trying to hold onto how things were when we had control, and when things made sense. "How things were" can easily be associated with "who I am" and the deeper identity question of "who will I become, and what will this mean?" as a result of this change. I found myself starting to enter this struggle without the vocabulary and the nous to know what it meant, and how to react. I wanted to hold on and, at the same time, my mind was often imagining the worst possible scenarios for catastrophic change. In darker moments, I imagined myself blind, helpless, alone, and even homeless. I felt vulnerable, and sorry for myself, and did not know what to do about it. It was a turbulent time of uncertainty, and the struggle between hope and fear in the space of that uncertainty was very much alive. If communication is one of the main ways that people manage and reduce uncertainly, as well as navigate change, then I knew it would be the key to understanding how I would work through the strange balancing act in which I now found myself.

During that summer of 2011, I began to perceive myself consciously holding onto things I enjoyed that were sight intensive activities. Partly, I think, particular interests and passions had helped define me as a person for a long time. They were part of how I saw myself and expressed my creativity, and partly I could not imagine letting those things, and the sighted "me" that they represented, go. I knew deep down that I might have to, but I did not want to, nor did I know what I would replace them with at this point. As I felt my eyes decline slightly in late summer and early fall, I began to revel in things that I enjoyed that enabled me to feel competent and connected to the things I had loved for many years. Creative and imaginative activities such as cooking, gardening, lapidary arts, music, and reading, became priorities for me because they might well be slipping away. That summer and into the fall, I had just a glimpse of the vision loss to come that I would have to adapt to. It was a bitter sweet time of enjoying things in the moment, and recognizing their more troubled and precarious place in my life story ahead.

August was sweetened considerably by my freedom from campus until the following August. I had bumped into Hema, a former colleague, at a grocery store in town several months ago and we had become friends. She wanted to get together for coffee and talk over ideas I might have for her to pursue a Ph.D., which we did. As we chatted, we shared where we were in our lives relationally. We talked about the complexity of the Indian—British historical and political relationship—not seeing it as a possible parallel or metaphoric conversation for ourselves at the time. We became friends over the next few months on a level we never did previously as colleagues. She even took me to my first eye test when this all began in May. Neither of us had any interest in each other romantically as colleagues and then friends, but things changed quickly. One day we kissed, we began to date, and soon we were inseparable. Soon I could not imagine life without her.

Holding On and Letting Go

I became mindful of enjoying and making the most of things that I had enjoyed for years, and that were part of me. In terms of cooking, for example, I enjoyed the fact that I could still drive to purchase the ingredients I needed. I could see the garlic and onions well enough to cut them up finely, and not cut my fingers. I could read the spice names and how much of each I was putting in. I could still see the oven settings, and read the oven clock with either eye, although I never really used the clock. The oven clock became one of the things I used regularly to check my sight in each eye—one eye, then the other, then both together. These were simple things that I had taken for granted up until now, and I had no idea when they would be difficult for me. Cooking represented my independence and the fact that I still had good enough vision for the simple tasks associated with feeding. Cooking also represented a sort of normalcy in the early stages of dating Hema in fall 2011. I enjoyed cooking for Hema. She cooked for me also, but now she was in a new job and I was home a lot with a much more flexible time schedule than she had. She would help sometimes, although I knew in reality I was always the sous chef—second to her in ability. She was a wonderful cook of her native south Indian food. If I was not careful she would take over in the kitchen, even if I was the primary cook for a particular dinner. We joked about this regularly.

A kitchen issue that did emerge had to do with where things such as utensils and containers were placed and stored. I started to get irritated when something was not where my hand expected them to be. Where had she put them? I worried that I would never find them now. This was odd and overly dramatic in that I could still see utensils and containers well. It was a small kitchen and things were never that difficult to find, so why was I annoyed and frustrated at the shifting placement of things? I had noticed that when I tell people I am experiencing vision problems, some of them listen and then turn around and expect you to be able to do all of the same things as normal. I was trying to say "please recognize that I need things to be where I expect them" I am not being over controlling or routinized as these insistences might normally be interpreted, I HAVE to insist on these adaptations to predictability. In reality, these struggles for placement were most likely a fusion of both the need to consider the future difficulty of seeing things, and the growing presence and decision making of Hema in what was my house for ten years before I met her. She was starting to assert her own ideas of where things should be, and I was reacting to this shift in territory as much as the vision issue, perhaps even more.

One evening I was watching a documentary about a blind American mountain climber who had taken blind children from Tibet (a culture in which people often ostracized blind children for apparently having sinned in a previous life) up some of the highest peaks in the Himalayan mountains. There was one moment in the story where he said that he is blind so needs to know where things are and how to put his hands on them. YES, I thought, he gets it! Whether in the Himalayas or my kitchen, the principle is the same—consistency reduces frustration, and minimizes relational conflict! At the same time I had to realize that I was not anywhere near being blind, as this inspiring mountain climber was. I would need to be more flexible and let go of the anxiety I was channeling into the issue of object placement, so that Hema was not walking on egg-shells in my home all of the time. This was the last thing I wanted. I knew that I also needed to learn to share what had been my single guy territory for some years.

I still loved my hobby of lapidary arts—cutting stones for jewelry. I had learned how to cut stones during my tenure year after a lifelong fascination with rocks and all things geological. I believed that partly inherited this from my mother who also loved rocks. I had needed a creative release from the grind of the last year or so of tenure-track life, and embracing the lapidary arts was a perfect relief. I could make something of beauty and, when the stone was finished, I could enjoy it or have it made into something for someone. Mum always wore something I had cut for her whenever I went home. I had put many of the stones I had cut over the years out onto a tray so that I could enjoy just looking at them. I reminisced about the times when I had purchased the rough rock material, or when I cut them. I wanted to continue to cut stones, although I had gravitated towards using magnifying glasses while cutting the stones. I had to take breaks I did not used to have to take, so that I could dry the stones and look really closely at them to make sure I was cutting them properly. I endured the frustration of making rookie mistakes like cutting flat spots on stones that should have been perfectly curved and smooth, but I enjoyed the pleasure of finishing more stones. I was already cutting the largest size on the metal templates I had—52 mm × 38 mm oval—which were, I believe, designed for belt buckles and really large bolo's and pendants, but I needed to be creative in this way for as long as I could. I still had a large box full of rocks to cut, and I wanted to keep going.

My mind sometimes wandered to the question of when I could no longer cut stones. Which would be the last stone I would cut, and for whom would I cut my last piece? What would it be like to sell or give away my machines and rocks? Another thing I had loved might well be stripped from me by this disease. But balancing the somewhat morbid thoughts and feelings of loss, I knew I would have to adapt and be creative in a different way when the time came. Perhaps my mind would be proactive in simply losing interest in rocks, which would make the loss much less painful.

Gardening also remained a passion for me. The summer of 2011 when I had been diagnosed, I grew an enormous crop of chili peppers. They were about the only thing besides figs that grew well in that long dry, hot summer. The bright summer light of that year was just beginning to bother my eyes. I loved to see the garden grow, but I had to shade from the sun very actively. My eyes began to shy away from the brightness. I began to organize outdoor activities such as gardening and walking around when the light was dimmest, and least painful. Hema helped me pick figs, and we made smoothies almost every day while the crop lasted. She helped me pick chilies in August and September. We cooked with them fresh, and I also roasted them in large batches to make bags full of home grown dried chilies, and chili powder. The roasting peppers filled the house with a beautiful aroma in early fall. We have a supply that should last at least for a year. As I picked the last of the peppers and pulled up the plants to go into the compost, I wondered if I would be gardening by the summer of 2012. I joked to myself that if I lost a lot of vision this year at least I would not have to look at all the weeds next year! At the same time would I need to move if gardening would become impossible for me. This was a big yard, and it required someone who could see well to take care of it all. To fight off these thoughts, I resolved to get the compost going again for next year, shredding leaves and adding whatever scraps from the kitchen we produced. I pressed on as normal—living as if things were going to be ok.

For several years I had played music casually with a couple of friends Steve and Art. Mostly I wrote the songs and we worked on them and played them together. It was a fun creative outlet for all of us. Sometimes we talked more than we played—supporting each other as we had when we were all department heads together a couple of years ago. It was a creative, nurturing, accepting environment we had created—largely without even really talking about it as such. It just evolved out of, and around, the shared creative activity. Although we did play at Art or my house occasionally, Steve's was a bigger, more band-friendly space in which to play. However, as the fall drew in, and the nights got darker, it became increasingly difficult for me to drive out to Steve's. They lived out near the country club golf course where there were no street lights. I had been to their house so many times but now, in the dark fall evenings, I had a hard time seeing where the driveway to their house was on the street. I began backing in so I could see ahead when I drove out of there later at night. I drove past it on several occasions. I stopped drinking while playing or driving completely. I needed the lights in the playing room just so. One evening the guys stated that if it would help we would play at my house and/or play one afternoon per week, so that it would be light for me coming and going. These were kind gestures, and I hoped to be playing and writing as close to normal as I could for as long as possible. I remained hopeful about music, if not so much the night driving involved. That fall we talked of a winter beach trip. It would be just the guys playing music and partying for a weekend. It would prove difficult to implement, but it was a nice assertion of our creative comradeship.

Reading was a central part of my life. I was an avid reader as a child. I remember walking to the Central Library in Bradford city center many times throughout my life growing up reading, borrowing book, enjoying browsing and just being around the stacks, even travelling there to do homework in happy schooldays of long ago. I dreamed of having a book of my own on one of the shelves one day. Reading and writing were, of course, integral to my work as a professor but, that fall, reading became difficult. I could use an e-reader and was fine reading on that. I had to wear both my regular glasses and magnification reading glasses on this early generation tablet, but I loved rereading all of the Sherlock Holmes adventures that fall. I read Rolling Stone magazine passed on to me by Steve, and the Guardian, passed on to me by Jon. But what would happen at the point I could not read even this way? Would I be disabled? Would I have to adapt to audio books and audio based technology for my job? Should I start this switch over to audio now I wondered? These were frightening prospects that were never far from the fearful back of my mind, and I never had anyone to ask for advice on these questions.

I was not a tech-savvy person at all, but I knew the technology was there to change to audio based "reading." I knew I should approach that as a natural transition from print, which was becoming increasingly difficult to read unless it was magnified at least 200%. Even with magnification, at least with WORD, the commands remained painfully small and unchanging. The scroll up and scroll down commands, for example, are tiny arrows and boxes which are pale blue on pale blue. I have jumped paragraphs many times writing this story when I wanted just to scroll a line or two. Also with a little ironic twist that I had never noticed before, I realized that although the zoom feature does help—I am now using 200%, the zoom command itself remains tiny! How come the zoom doesn't zoom?! Perhaps there's a "low vision" version of WORD I can use? I would need to look into this sometime.

I realized that it was important to stay positive, and keep things in perspective. I remember waking up one morning, checking both of my eyes on objects around the bedroom, and happily telling myself: "Today I can read, today I can drive, today I can recognize my sweetheart's face!"

Other mornings I would playfully name other things I could still do. I would do this occasionally to reinforce that I was still more or less ok.

Falling Back—Flipping Forward

In the beginning of November 2011, right around the time when daylight savings time ends and the clocks "fall back" an hour, something started to change for me. I was doing alright up until this point but, with the ushering in of the darker side of the year, I was beginning to have difficulties. I was just over a month away from the first six month check-up and I had had no pain up until now, when I started to feel dizziness and a headache. I went with Hema one evening to PF Chang's, which she really liked. The place was so dark I could not read the menu. I found this disturbing. I could not see very well, and the lack of light was making me feel nauseous and depressed. I managed the feelings somehow by controlling where my eyes went. If I kept my eyes on the table right in front of me, I was ok. If I tried to look around the restaurant, my eyes got overstimulated, and bad feelings came rushing at me like being sea sick. I felt compelled to get out of there as soon as I could. Hema was understanding but wanted a nice long dinner on this relaxed Thursday evening. I could not stand just sitting there, and had a hard time explaining why to her. I tried, but it was not working for some reason. She went to the rest room after eating, and I told her I would wait outside as soon as I had paid for dinner. I could not wait to get out of there. I sat on the bench outside and, looking at the ground just in front of me, I sucked in as much fresh cold air as I could. I felt awful, but this helped. I felt like I was on the cold deck of a roiling ferry, still sea sick but the fresh air was a lifesaver that I clung to.

The next morning I called the office of my retina specialist. I explained who I was and that I was feeling light headed, dizzy, and that I was having a hard time feeling good in dim lighting. The office technician told me that the problem would not be related to my eye condition, and that I might want to see my primary care physician. I believed it was my eyes, but she did not. I asked if I could move my appointment up by a month and she said no, we would stick to the six month check-up time in December. I asked her if she thought it might be blood pressure related and she said that is what she would have thought it might be. I rushed over to my primary care physician's office. In retrospect I should have called for a specific appointment but, being inexperienced in the routines of health care, I did not. I asked for a blood pressure test. At this point it was creeping into early Friday afternoon, and I could tell the energy in the doctor's office was waning significantly. The nurse who did my test was not friendly or particularly caring. I could tell she was ready for the weekend. She told me: "No your blood pressure is fine so it ain't that"

"Well can I see Dr. Little anyway?" I asked, "Just to figure out what's going on?"

"No, well you'd have to call and make an appointment for that" she said indifferently. But I am already here I thought to myself. I would have to call the office from inside the office?!

"Is he available this afternoon?" I asked, hopeful that she would help me.

"No there's nothing available, you'd have to call" she dismissed.

She continued, "And If you're having a heart attack or something urgent, go to the ER or Urgent care, don't come here ... some of 'em do you know!" she said wryly as if inviting me in to make fun of people.

Wow! I thought to myself, I have spent most of a Friday running around and waiting around for this. I had no answers and did not know where to go. The callous sarcasm of the nurse stuck in my mind. If I was in a life threatening condition I needed to know what to do. I must have caught these people on a bad Friday. My heart went out to all the other people who had gone to the wrong place in need, and suffered the consequences. And, I was rapidly developing an ever deepening sense of empathy to the elderly who spend much of their time in and between medical appointments patiently waiting. I left for home with nothing accomplished. I knew I needed to get smarter about where to be for what was wrong, but when you are not sure what is wrong, it is hard to know where to begin!

I was playing music that weekend and explained my health care experience to Steve who encouraged me to try spending some time outside in the light. He thought that I may be reacting to the ending of daylight savings and the onset of the darker fall/winter environment. The next day I spent time in the yard soaking in some daylight, albeit with my eyes well covered, and it did make a difference. I also began taking a vitamin D supplement, thinking at least part of what I was experiencing might have been a touch of seasonal affect disorder. I never really knew what it was, but I still believe it was something to do with my eyes changing.

I soon felt much brighter. At the same time, I was also experiencing noticeable vision problems in my right eye. I could tell things were more difficult to see clearly. Faces on television through my right eye were becoming frighteningly distorted. I resolved to stick to the six month check-up as they had advised me, despite Hema prompting me to try again to change it. I told her that they would not change it. I believed that they really needed the full six months as a yardstick from the first diagnosis. Perhaps it had more to do with the fact that they did not think that what I was experiencing was related to the cone-dystrophy. Perhaps not, but in the back of my mind I remember reading that complications can arise and lead to other condition. The month or so around November, just before my next appointment, would bring deterioration of my vision and new things to adapt to.

One chilly fall evening we went to see a play production at the community college where Hema was teaching. It was hard work for me to look at the faces of the actors on stage for the duration of the play and try to figure out what they were trying to communicate. Their faces were almost like blank ovals in the distance. My eyes were tired by the end of the play. Driving back home afterwards with Hema, I sat quietly wondering if I could have driven the thirty minutes or so across town if I really had to. I thought that I could, as I always managed to in life, but I was glad I did not have to. I had given night time driving duties—especially in places where she was more familiar—more or less over to Hema. It was unusual. I usually drove, and was clearly having a hard time relinquishing control to her. As a result I was quick, if mostly gentle, to point out her bad driving habits.

"If that truck had decided to come into this turn lane it would have been your fault. Wait until the line for the left turn lane appears" I said a little sternly.

I know I also commonly told her she was drifting in the lane which she usually acknowledged that she does. This night she listened and allowed me the luxury of advising her—even though it was something I would have a difficult time receiving myself. Was I becoming the expert who cannot do it himself? I found myself checking both eyes, trying to read things like gas station signs that used to be easy, to see if I could define any changes. I was giving myself a constant letter test! The check-up meeting was still a month away (December 16th) and it did feel like there had been some more rapid loss. It was hard to know who to talk to about all of this, I thought to myself as we drove home. Again I thought that some sort of vision loss coach would have been useful in helping me understand things, and keeping things in perspective, but there was not one that I knew of.

I was visiting Hema one early winter evening. She lived in a gated apartment community so she gave me the gate code: #1755. I drove up to the pad and typed in the code. Nothing happened. I tried it again, and it started ringing someone's apartment or cell phone. I tried again and could not get it to work. I could not quite see the keys, so I guessed, based on their location in a square of 10 digits. One will be the top left; seven will be bottom left and five in the middle of the pack, I told myself. Maybe I pressed star instead of pound? I could not tell from the dim light. Try again. Someone pulled in behind me, which made fiddling around with the pad uncomfortable as I was keeping them waiting, so I drove around and away to let them through. I was agitated and angry. The pad was unlit. "Could they not put a fucking light on the key pad?" I said to myself, angrily. How was I supposed to see the keys? I pulled over near the community office and was angry, and expressed this to Hema when I called for help. She never liked me cursing but I was angry, and just venting. I was not blaming her in any way. Perhaps at the same time I was also afraid. Everyone else seemed to get through the key pad barrier ok but, for me, the pad was missing a much needed light. I would have to start bringing a flashlight, or chance that I could sneak in behind another car, or take my chances with whatever light there happened to be near the pad. Instead of getting angry, especially with Hema, why could I not break problems like this down into practical strategies for easily getting through the situation? After all, even if I could not get through the gate, her apartment was only a short walk on the other side of the pedestrian gate? Being unable to drive through the gate was not the end of the world. Was I angry at the key pad, the people who did not bother lighting it, my bad luck, or simply at my eyes for letting me down? I would need to think through these situational layers more effectively if I was going to keep things in perspective, and adapt practically to the reality of lower vision.

When I did drive, I had asked Hema to clearly tell me what to do while driving, turn here, get in the left lane, and so on. She did give me directions even when it was obvious what I needed to do, which was good. This helped us avoid judgment calls while driving based on what might or might not be obvious to me. We both knew that ambiguity would cause problems. However, it was still a difficult adjustment for me and, sometimes, I snappily corrected her directions, and got annoyed, as she was telling me the very things I had asked her to do—direct me, even if it seemed obvious. I know she also felt tense when I was driving, and I would need to accept her directions. It was not that I resented the directions, rather, I felt vulnerable and angry that I needed them in the first place. But, I was putting her in a classic no-win situation—direct me and get snapped at, or miss a direction and get snapped at. This was something else I would need to work on in terms of communicating difficult emotions effectively.

Besides switching my role as primary driver with Hema—especially at night—and becoming the reluctant back seat driver, I began to reorganize my everyday life in ways that minimized the work that my eyes had to do. I was protecting the eye sight that I did still have. Normally in relationships I realize that there is a to and fro around issues of constancy and change. Few people want to be with someone who is dogmatic about things being done a specific way all of the time. Similarly the energy and fun of a relationship comes from being open to each other's ideas for how to do things, and how to do things differently. Simply, there is a normal interplay of comforting stability and energizing change. Adapting to a different set of expectations about the relative dynamics of stability and change based on my eye problems would become a stressor for us—something that we would have to become mindful of. Hema is naturally a change-oriented person. She is interested in coaching, and loves to do simple things such as driving to the store and so on differently—sometimes for the sake of the difference, and sometimes just to see if there is a better way. I had also prided myself on being change oriented. I had taught change related courses many times. I had been a department head for 8 years and pushed changes to the department constantly. I changed my styles; tastes; home decor, and so, on, as a regular part of who I was, and how I lived. However, things quickly began to change for me in ways that made me want to hold on. The need I felt to protect my eyes had begun to shift my orientation. Conflicts arose when normal expectations of change clashed often quite momentarily, and never in a relationally threatening way, with my emerging need for predictability and control of my visual environment.

I began to notice that street signs, even highway signs, were far too small. Why were signs and highways so small, and so badly lit in the US, I now often wondered? Perhaps it was because there are just so many more miles to cover with lights here versus smaller European countries, or it was just less of a priority. I had navigation on my smart phone but had not gotten into using it yet, preferring to work out directions with Hema as needed, and avoiding driving where I was unfamiliar.

Another example of this need for unusual levels of control had to do with computer use. Hema loved to check her email when she was at my house. She would log out of my Hotmail and log into hers, and then check her messages. Whether she logged out or left me to do that, the page size was back to normal (100%) after she used it. This began to irk me and I reached a point where I would get angry and tell her not to use my computer unless she put the page size back to 200%—a size where I could still comfortably work. At 100% I would struggle, and it was unnecessary work for my eyes to find the small commands to change it back to 200%.

There were many other micro-level ways that these stressors expressed themselves and were dealt with by us during these early adaptive and sense-making days. At times these issues were reframed by Hema in ways that made sense to her, but which were not the point I was trying to make. For example, she resolved to "work on me" in terms of my openness to change:

"Hey take this road home to my place. See, its less lights, and about five minutes less driving for you." She tried to persuade me.

"No thanks, its way out in dark country roads, and I like to stick to the main roads I know. The main road is well lit and I know where the stop lights and turns are." I responded trying to show her why I was doing what I was doing.

"But just try this way …" she would try again sometimes …

She definitely meant well. And who wants to be with someone who does the same things the same ways all of the time, and who gets irritable if they are changed? But this was for me not a personality issue, but one of minimization of eye work, and control of the risks associated with being in less certain driving conditions. Driving was, for me now, about destination—getting there safely and with minimal stress and eye fatigue. It was much less these days about the journey itself.

I do not know that we talked about these dialectical and adaptive issues that well initially. Much of the time it was me getting upset, and Hema accommodating, which was not healthy either. She did tell me I was short tempered with her at times. The question did occur to me: Were we simply reproducing an unequal relationship through these practices? I have to say that I believe that they were genuine reactions and responses to fear and uncertainty, as well as ways of marking the need to rethink expectations and reorganize around my progressive vision loss. At the same time, I was conscious that she had been abused and taken for granted by her first husband who, by all accounts, except his of course, had taken advantage of her kind and accommodating nature and persona as an Indian woman. Neither of us wanted to recreate this nightmare. At the same time, I needed a little more predictability and control of my environment but it would have to be just that—motivated by and organized around my progressive vision loss, not any desire to have a submissive and accommodating woman constantly adapting to my whims.

In these early stages of the disease, I was preparing for the unknown—pre-grieving—for a time when I would not be able to do the things I could do now, and I would not be able to be the person I am now, at least in the same way. But at this point, I had no idea how quickly the disease would move. I had no idea "how long I had" as one friend, Molly Miller, questioned me. The question stuck with me. It made the process, the journey, whatever this was, a finite thing. I would be there someday—a different person, unable to see except with peripheral vision. I was afraid, and did not know how to adapt given the uncertainty vacuum surrounding my disease. At times it felt like I was preparing for a character I was about to play, and that I did not really need to be this structured or serious about things yet. I was also asserting a need for Hema and myself to take the disease seriously. It was not an acting job, it was a real story we were in as the main characters. For now, I was enjoying the things I had enjoyed for much of my life while adapting to the difficulty of continuing to engage in these predominantly visual activities.

At this early point in the story I was anxious, shocked, and confused. I wanted to retreat to the familiar—to tell myself that things were still normal. Part of this emotional reaction comes from imagining the worst—a life without vision and all of the loss, vulnerability, and uncertainty associated with that. Part of the imagining of loss, for me had to do with the deep interruption to my sense of self and my life story. Who would I be—who would I become? This narrative interruptus represented, for me, the possibility of having to spend much of my life struggling to find new ways to express myself and live. On a deeper thematic level, it also represented a sort of crisis of independence. I had always viewed myself as an independent person. I had come to America alone, and found my own way to what I wanted to do. I enjoyed my single life for many years, and so on. Of course, I was intimately connected to the help and friendship of others along the way, but the independent streak I enjoyed seeing in myself was a central archetype of my own life story up until now. Would I need to completely revise how I narrated my life from this point forward and, if so, what storylines were out there ready for me to piece together into my story going forward? If I had choices, what were they, and how much choice would I have over them? What were the archetypes of the stories of blind people? These were questions I did not want to wrestle with but I knew I had no choice. I knew I could not live in the—albeit sweet—denial of assuming that things would essentially always stay the same.

This question of how people narrate their experience of vision loss, and how this changed their life stories, would be a very important question for me to come back to later. At this point, I was conscious of a sort of narrative pressure to have something like a positive transformational turn, and I did not feel it at all at this point. I was far from feeling heroic. I did not want to be told to "be positive" or "think positive." These seemed like trite clichés spoken by people who were not going through the same experience. I did not want to be fake about where I was in my own story. At the same time this pressure told me that this positive turn was one of the narrative archetypes that were valued culturally here in America. It was a way forward through the narrative interruptus or disruption of disease based trauma that people understood and admired.

By way of a parallel case, we were at the end of the Iraq war, and towards the end of the Afghan wars, and CNN was regularly showing disabled veterans coming home without legs or arms, and with a host of other massively traumatic injuries. They were shown to be turning their lives into inspiring success stories. These success stories were aired to motivate others, and show that character, determination, and patriotism can overcome all obstacles. These stories were often immensely moving. Like many of us I was filled with admiration for their courage, but were these stories the norm, or were they cherry picked for their newsworthiness and affirmation of nationalistic as well as human values? On some level this was "war journalism." How many of their beautiful life partners actually stuck with them and helped them through everything as they did in the news stories? Could I live up to these lessons of inspirational courage, or would I end up with a different response to the loss I would experience? Would I have a loser story?! I was not a legless but determined Special Olympics swimming hopeful who somehow turned their terrible landmine injury into an opportunity for success. What would be *my* story, indeed my narrative choices in moving beyond my own trauma? I simply did not know, but I knew at this point that the images of such courage were more anxiety provoking, even depressing, for me than inspirational. They filled me with more questions that I found uncomfortable. How did the legless swimmer get to the pool every day? Was he able to have sex? How many people were inspired by him, and how many pitied him, or even made fun of him? The cable news clips always seemed to round off these jagged story edges, and fill in any gaps that might evoke questions. Plus, I simply wanted to cling to the things I loved, and find a way to hang onto the activities, and the meanings they represented for me, for as long as I could.

One hopeful turn in my thinking happened in that late fall when I began to wonder what form of creativity and expression might emerge once all of the hobbies and familiar activities I had loved were slowly stripped away from me. Would some form of expression that is grounded in one of the other senses come through and surprise me, or was this based on a mythology about blind people? Would I find new activities to occupy my time? Would I be useful to others in some new way? Would losing my sight be a "blessing in disguise" in some unforeseeable way as many motivational speakers and heroic news stories might have me believe?

To counterbalance this hopeful turn, my mind also wandered into the darker questions of what would happen to me. Would I have to have special living arrangements? If so when? Would I be able to keep my job? Could I still be successful as a professor without being able to see well or at all, or would I just be hanging on, and in the way? Would I be hopeless, maybe even homeless? My friend and staff member Gloria once told me that we were all just a few steps from the streets, and I wondered if I was walking those steps. Who, if anyone, would take care of me—given that Hema was my only "family" here in the US? The worry over basic mechanics was never far from me. The communicative art of balancing the hopes and the fears would become crucial "health" issue for me, but it was not proving to be an easy art to master.

Central to this balance was the blessing of supportive communication. "I don't want you to worry. I want you to hold your head up high and always be positive" Hema's words helped many times during difficult moments when my mind wandered to the dark possibilities ahead for me—for us.

Just before my next appointment in December, I was coming out of the post office one day—dropping off Christmas cards for people back home. As I walked towards my car I saw someone coming towards me, but his face was completely blank. I knew he was a man but I had no idea what his facial features were, if I knew him or not, or what his facial expression was. On top of the horror of distorted faces, now I was seeing blank faces. The image stopped me in my tracks. I was frozen for a moment between hope and deep, deep worry. I shook off the moment as best I could, and walked on into the season of hope. Billy Idol's haunting lyric, "eyes without a face …" popped into my mind, and the song stayed with me.

· 3 ·

FIRST INJECTION

December 23rd 2011

Bud:	"I will pray for you my friend"
Pete:	"And I will pray for you"
Bud:	"We always did make a good team"
Pete:	"Yes, we did, and we're both still in the game …"
	(Excerpt from a Facebook conversation with Bud Goodall (Kellett, 2013)

I went back for my six month check up on December 19th 2011. They did lots of tests and, when I met Dr. Sanders after the test data had been collected, he was concerned and puzzled. He asked me how my sight felt and I told him that I thought the right eye had declined. He told me that he was seeing something odd develop in the right eye, and that I would need to come back for more tests as soon as possible. They would need more information before deciding what to do. Quickly the discussion had shifted from a routine check-up to a serious investigation. The hope I had that this would just be something we monitored every six months, and that I would be fine, was quickly shifting into something very different. It was Friday and he asked me to come back as soon as possible. I made an appointment to come back on December 23rd—just a few days from then. I was anxious and fearful and yet I wanted to get to the 23rd and find out what was happening. I was glad we decided to stay in and around Greensboro for the Christmas season so we could begin treatment if necessary. What follows is a description of the first injection I had.

It was the day before Christmas Eve—10:30 Friday morning Dec 23rd when I returned. I could tell that the doctor's office staff members were antsy to get their Christmas photo done and be off on their breaks starting at noon. I could not blame them. They all probably had lots to do. Also, working with eye issues had to be somewhat dull, if meaningful work. Eye patients often do not respond communicatively the same way other types of patients might. In the waiting room they were often silently hunched over, with big patches over their eyes—the "post-ops" from Thursday's surgeries. Friday mornings seemed to be quiet and serious in the waiting room. Usually there was just the slightly annoying trickle of the water feature, and the background murmur of the office staff making appointment reminder calls for next week, and processing patients. We mostly just waited for our names to be called. This morning the waiting room was full with post-ops as they were trying to get people checked before the Christmas break. I quickly realized I would have a long wait that day.

We completed several more tests, including a color recognition/blindness test. My performance on the color test was a surprise. I did not realize how much color differentiation I had lost in the right eye. With the left eye, I got almost all of the number and letter recognition tests correct. With the right eye I only got a few correct. I had no idea. I had noticed that the green of the stop signs had shifted a little towards a more blue-green, but overall I had significantly overestimated my color acuity. Color blindness was apparently beginning to creep in quite subtly. This also made me realize that one's own perceptions of one's vision can be unreliable. It is easy not to notice the small creeping changes, and the brain learns to ignore the gaps, and go with what information it does get from the eyes. We moved through to the photography room for more tests.

After several blasts of photographs through my dilated eyes Matt, the genial technician, had me curl my toes for a few minutes to help dilate my eyes enough to get a good picture. The nurse pumped the dye into my arm quicker than last time—it made me really nauseas for a second, at which point the tech assured me that this does happen in a small number of patients. It was nothing to worry about. Perhaps the speedy injection was part of the push to get done by noon? I had waited a while to be seen and noon was creeping ever closer.

I had read somewhere that Cone Dystrophy is often associated with other "complications" of the retinas. The article I read did not specify anything beyond this fact. My mind came back to this as Dr. Sanders explained to me that I was experiencing a swelling of the right retina that is causing a "puckering" of the retina. This could explain the awful horror movie-like distortions and blankness I had been experiencing as I looked at people's faces both live and on television. I had to train myself to not move my eyes a certain way while looking at faces, or they would appear as an awful caricature. The people I was looking at of course did not know this unless I told them, so who knows what they thought when I averted my gaze from their faces. Looking slightly to the left of people made their faces appear normal again. I was instinctively trying to find some good retina with which to process the image. His diagnosis also explained the fuzziness and vision loss I felt I had experienced since the last visit. He gave me the choice to wait until after the holidays or begin treatment immediately. He was clear that if I waited I might well experience further irreparable vision loss. He had urgency in his voice as he encouraged me to go ahead and start treatment now. We ran quickly through the waiver form. He stressed several times that this was not a cure, but a potentially effective treatment in stopping further decline. We both agreed to start immediately, and we were quickly into the process of preparing me for administering the injections. It was a relief to be starting an actual course of treatment, but I shuddered slightly when he responded to my question about whether the injections were *in the eye*: "Yes, in the eye, but we numb the eye with an injection before the medication so you won't feel much of anything" he assured me.

I swallowed nervously, as I now realized I would be getting two injections in my right eye. I tried not to visualize what was coming.

"Did you put the Avastin away?" Dr. Sanders asked the nurse.

Yeees! The nurse responded, stretching the word out into a gentle whine—probably wishing for noon and the start of the holidays.

"Well, we have to start this now" said Dr. Sanders.

I was the last soul in the place, holding everybody up from their office Christmas picture and lunch on the boss, or whatever they had planned. The nurse technician numbed my eye. Just a few minutes later Dr. Sanders came in and, again, explained the injection procedure. Even worse than the injections, was having my eyelid clipped open so that I could not blink my right eye lid. It felt very vulnerable, and I was frightened. My eye was numbed with the first injection which did hurt a little. Then, a little later, the main needle with the Avastin was inserted. I had been directed to watch the nurse as she waved her fingers off to my left. He came at my eye from the other side so, mercifully, I never saw a needle coming at me, and actually felt very little physically. All the while he encouraged me; telling me I was safe and that I was doing a great job. There really was not much to it physically. I was done quickly. By the time I had finished making my next appointment, the staff had gathered around Dr. Sanders for their festivities. It was a happy scene, and I slipped away to enjoy the season as much as I could.

Walking outside with Hema we decided to have tea somewhere on the nearby State Street. It was a nice idea, in theory, to have somewhere to go afterwards. Neither of us had been in that area in a long time, and perhaps we might see some last minute gift for Christmas for someone. But it was a mistake. It was a painfully bright day to walk around with dilated eyes. We did have tea at a café, although it was very difficult for me to see the menu and choose the tea. There was even a Santa Claus sitting outside one store wishing people well. However it was so painfully sunny and bright that day that I could not wait to get home and just close the blinds. I followed her in my car and, once home, stayed inside in the safe dimness for the rest of the day. This would be the post-injection day ritual from now on—get home to the safety of the shadows.

That afternoon I was home alone and the engagement ring I had ordered for Hema arrived—just in time! It was soon to get engaged after only a few months but I knew she was the person I wanted to be with, and I wanted to buy her something really special that she could enjoy. I also wanted to buy her a ring when I could see it well enough to enjoy it myself, sparkling on her finger. I would give it to her the next evening—Christmas eve. A week or so ago I had insisted on decorating the Christmas tree myself, just to know that I could do it. Hema misunderstood this as me not wanting her to be involved, which was not my intent at all. Later that evening of the 23rd we sat with just the tree lights on and, although the twinkling lights dazzled my eyes, it felt good just to be home with special presents under the tree, a special person next to me, and the surreal drama of the day behind us.

Checking in on Facebook the next morning I read an excerpt of a critical article by Chris Hedges posted by Bud Goodall: "A nation that destroys its systems of education, degrades its public information, guts its public libraries and turns its airwaves into vehicles for cheap, mindless amusement becomes deaf, dumb and blind. It prizes test scores above critical thinking and literacy …"

I was irate, especially that someone avowing liberal policy and critique would use "deaf, dumb, and blind" in this way. I rarely post opinion on Facebook but this time I posted, "Yes, but can we stop using deaf, dumb, and blind as pejoratives?"

I began to notice language use such as this much more, and it bothered me that we use blind when we mean someone cannot, or chooses not to, perceive something. Being deaf or blind is different from choosing not to perceive something. Being unable to speak is not the same as being stupid. I doubt that many would disagree with me but these word uses were deeply ingrained culturally. This was a cultural struggle over language and meaning that I had never noticed before. No one responded to my post, not even a single "like" which made me wonder if I had overreacted. I noticed a few days after the injection that my right eye had begun to improve slightly. Faces were no longer terribly distorted. Could this wild card of an off-label medication actually be working? My mind had set itself on the idea that I was heading inevitably towards the strange and very scary world of blindness, but I now also had considerable hope. This might just work.

We spent New-year's at the beach—beginning a tradition for us. I insisted on driving the four hours both there and back. It felt really good to do that successfully. I was fine as long as she read the road signs for me. On the morning of new-year's day Hema got us up before dawn. We made hot tea and bundled up on the balcony from where we could see far out to sea. We took pictures every few minutes of the dawn as it emerged into daybreak by 7:15 am or so. The pictures were beautiful, and the getaway was just what we both needed after the stress of the diagnosis and start of treatment. It would be a new year filled with taking pleasure in the things I could see, and so much more. Perhaps some of these things, like a simple sunrise over the ocean, I would see in a different—more appreciative—light this year, and be a better person for it.

The trip sparked further discussion of travel plans. Hema dreamt of taking me to the Caribbean, although I told her, only half-jokingly, that somewhere overcast and gloomy would be much better for me. Bright sunshine was hard for me to take anymore. We would adjust based on this. As we talked, we decided that we would visit England this summer, and also see some of her native India. That would be an ambitious trip. I wanted to see the Smithsonian gem and mineral collection again. She wanted to visit DC and also New York. We wanted to visit particular friends around the world. Part of me wondered if we were also unconsciously developing a sort of blind man's "bucket-list"—things to see before you cannot see anymore. Still, it was good for both of us to talk into reality our shared dreams. Most of the time Hema talked about her very specific dreams, and I simply listened, or talked in vague generalities—sometimes this was a source of frustration for her.

Learning to Share My Story So Far

"I'd give you one of mine if I could" —Dad

In these early stages I was very selective in choosing to whom I disclosed my condition. As I told my eighty year old father of the experience of the first injections he was shocked, and told me that I could have one of his eyes. I was deeply touched and thanked him for the gesture, and assured him that I would be alright. My younger brother, with whom I am close, assured me that there was no family history of the disease, and that he was sure I would be ok. I had to tell him again that, family history or not, it had definitely been diagnosed and we were "in treatment." He was surprised, thinking it not possible to have something like this happen to his brother. My twin brother told me he would rather live in denial than get tested for it to see if he had the same genetic mutation. He had been through so much with cancer that I did not blame him. My older brother told me that I needed to demand whatever treatments there were available. "Be aggressive in your own treatment" was his big brotherly message. I would come to understand that he was right.

Colleagues I was close to either did not know how to react, were sympathetic, and/or simply changed the subject. Others took the sharing of bad news as an opportunity to share their own troubles either empathically or occasionally in a selfish way—an opportunity to talk about themselves. On rare occasions, I did sense that the person I was telling was mostly relieved that it was not happening to them. This particular predatory disease had not thinned them out from the herd! Perhaps this instinctive relief partly explains why people are drawn to bad news and so many murder-based television shows. Oddly, often the people who changed the subject, or who seemed not to know how to react, were the ones who followed up later with requests for updates. All of this made me question how I reacted to peoples troubles when they have shared them with me. Looking back I do not think I did enough to communicate that I cared either time that my twin brother battled with cancer. I recognized that it was as hard for others to know how to react to my news now, as it was for me when my brother announced his cancer. It is difficult to know how to react, and how to communicate care, when you cannot really empathize completely, and you also do not want to say the wrong thing.

My close friend, Bud Goodall who is currently (at the end of 2011) fighting the fight of his own life with stage 4 pancreatic cancer, and who is remaining resolutely positive about it all—turning it once again as he does into an "ethnographic opportunity" told me to "rely on family, friends, and prayer." The first two I would have imagined him saying, but the third one was a surprise. Mortality does strange, and perhaps sometimes good things to all of us. I hoped Bud would be around for a long, long time. He is an inspiration to so many. His own life threatening situation enabled us to re-connect around health in a new way, and he was a constant encouragement to me while he was alive.

It was interesting, and revealing, to see each person I shared my condition with react from where and who they were in their own lives, and in terms of their relationship to me, and their ability to communicate care and concern.

Last spring semester, ironically just before my diagnosis in May, I had a blind student in my class—Kolby Garrison. She was a great student who taught me so much about the experience of living in a visual world as a blind person. Both she and her dog Sunny are Facebook friends, as well as real life friends now. I had no idea during that spring that she would come back into my life now as a source of great support and valuable information about blindness. I remember one day asking the class to turn with me to such and such page in the "purple book"—she stopped me and said she did not know what purple was! She had never seen it. How would you describe purple to someone who has never seen colors? I had her play the voice on her audio translation unit for me one day, and I was amazed at how quickly she could listen. The audio was going at, what was for me, lightning speed. It was far faster than I could have imagined or have followed. Just as sighted people can speed read, so she can speed listen.

I contacted her on Facebook a few months after the semester and asked if we could talk. I needed to seek out advice, common experience, and connection. In that very first conversation with Kolby she showed genuine interest in helping and advising me. We joked about her being on my "support team" as I went through this experience. She asked me about where I was in terms of vision loss and diagnosis. We shared notes on how little research there seems to be, and how there seems to be so little help in understanding how to adjust and live as a person with visual impairment or blindness. She told me that the doctors will advise nothing on this and she shared how frustrating it was for her when they were "trying" different medications and treatments—searching for something that might work for her years ago. We shared common frustrations. We resolved to stay in touch, which we did. She asked me if I had a girlfriend, and I said yes. She told me that it was common for partners to end relationships with people who develop vision problems. I was shocked by this and felt fortunate to talk to such a bright light as Kolby, and to have Hema standing by me. To be rejected relationally because one is losing one's sight must be unimaginably painful.

The new-year for me brought on a period of "putting my house in order." I wanted to move some assets over to Hema in the event of my death, which I did. I did a major clear out of my house and garden shed. I was putting things straight and making sure Hema would be ok financially if I died. I was not in any life threatening danger, but it made me feel more comfortable to make sure she was taken care of, if I could not take care of her. I wanted to take care of her, as much as she was taking care of me. My vision loss was nagging at me in terms of whether I would be able to give her what she wanted in life. It was a hollow, sad, disappointed feeling at times. Mostly, I would say, the feeling I had in darker moments was deep disappointment.

The Cone Dystrophy was just the beginning of an ever deepening mystery centered at the back of my eyes. At this point, as far as I knew anyway, I had two diseases at work in my eyes. Bulls-eye Cone Dystrophy (BCD) and now Wet Macular Degeneration (WMD) in what they call a non-age related form. I had no real understanding of the relationship between the two, other than that the Macular Degeneration seemed to be a complication of the Cone Dystrophy. I still did not know how one lead to the other, or why the Cone Dystrophy began in the first place. I do not know that anyone really knew.

· 4 ·

SECOND INJECTION

January 20th 2012

Hopeful Communication

At the next appointment on Friday 20th January 2012 I felt that I could read down further than last time on the eye chart that they use as a comparison point each time I go. Matt, the technician, did not say much, but I asked him for the results of the letter test anyway. He told me that, yes, I had gotten down on the size chart 2 levels further than last time in both eyes. I wondered why both eyes would improve when I had medication only in one. He explained that the left probably had to compensate less for the right, as it had improved. They worked together in ways I never knew before. I was thrilled inside, although such positives tend to get muted a little in the sometimes slow drag between rooms, and the different tests.

After just two bright retina pictures, I waited patiently for Dr. Sanders to hear and see the results. He popped round the door to say he would be with me in a minute. Probably a good sign—he wanted to share the positive moment with me. He came into the room and said he was excited to see me come back to find out how the first round of treatment had gone. He was bubbly with excitement. He wanted me to own the positive news, so he asked me how I thought the month had gone. I was much less bubbly, but shared that I though the right eye had improved and that it felt that things had "sort of settled down, yeah settled down" meaning I could not detect the sometimes daily lessening of sight I had experienced at times before we started with the injections. It was a good feeling. He showed me the images from before (a month ago) and today. The reduction in swelling both in the image based picture and the numbered chart, were very clear and encouraging. We shared a happy moment and a resolve to see the process through the four injections, and possibly on to less frequent injections after that. It was a really good hope filled visit.

Finally, I mentioned to Dr. Sanders that I was thinking of getting some transitions lenses to help with the often difficult transition of bright and dim light between indoors and outdoors, particularly on campus where we are in and out of buildings all day. He told me not to buy any expensive glasses yet until we know what is happening. This brought home the uncertainty of his expectations for the process, and tempered the moment slightly but, overall, we were both happy with the results.

I drove home thankful not only for the good news, but for the slight cloud-cover that made driving less painful. I wore two layers of sun glasses to block out the glare and drove carefully, defensively, and uneventfully straight home to the safe shadows.

When the numbing shot wore off, I was left with some pain in the eye, though not as much as the very dramatic redness might suggest. I felt for a few days like I had been punched in the eye. I looked like I had been strangled hard enough to burst the blood vessels in my eye. I felt a tinge of pity as I looked at my face. It must have been a shock to others to see me. Much worse than the redness (sub-conjunctival hemorrhage) was the terrible cold/flu symptoms and the slight feeling of choking I had for a day or two. My tongue felt big and dry. It seemed as though I had caught a cold immediately after the injection, but these were clearly side effects. This immune system vulnerability was something that my twin brother lived with constantly as a result of two rounds of near death with Hodgkin's Lymphoma. For me, this was a temporary symptom. But for him, it was something he lived with as a constant threat as he rode in and out of London to work on public transportation amidst the grime, germs, and viruses of others. This was a small price to pay for me to have a chance of holding off vision loss. Probably for him, also, his vulnerability was small price to pay in his mind for being alive. Sadly, we never talked on this level but, perhaps, my own current brush with decline and mortality was bringing on a deeper feeling of empathy with him which I did not-*could not*-feel at the time.

Because the side effects were so much worse this time, I decided to go back and re-read the published side effects lists for Avastin. Side effects were not something that was discussed with the doctor. He told me that I would have some redness in the eye and that if there was anything else that came up—to let them know. The literature provided at the doctor's office mentioned that some life threatening reactions/complications have occurred in a very small number of patients. These include strokes and heart attacks. So far, thankfully, I had not had any indicators of these, and it seemed that many lists of side effects routinely include these. I had also beaten the odds on gastrointestinal issues associated with vomiting and constipation. I had not developed an eye infection. Given all of this, I was feeling quite fortunate. I did get the subconjunctival hemorrhage (bloodshot eye), common cold, and the slight tongue and throat swelling. But, overall, my experience was in concert with the doctors literature, which positively framed taking the medication against some slight risk of side effects and starker reality of not taking the drug … "Without treatment, vision loss may be quick and severe." Perhaps it is normal psychologically to believe you might beat the odds on the list of side effects? Perhaps it would work for me without terrible results? I certainly hoped that it would.

My sweetheart came over that first night with lots of food from one of our favorite places. At my request she had made sure there was no MSG used in the cooking. This one chemical I was being treated with felt powerful and difficult enough through these side effects for now, and MSG always had a strange impact on me—agitating my brain. As she walked in she looked at my eye and sensed my fragility as I probably carried these side effects heavily perhaps dramatically at first. She began to cry. Weeks later she told me that that night I looked "pitiful."

"What's wrong?" I asked.

"I just want you to be alright. I just want you to be alright?" she sobbed into my chest. I held her and told her the good news, and clarified that this looked a lot worse than it felt, and not to worry. I told her I wanted a celebration whiskey. She was hesitant—working on the assumption, probably true, that this was not a good combination either. The day before, I had picked up from the office a book that just came out in which I have a chapter. Unfortunately, the print was so small I could not easily read the chapter, but it still felt good to see my name and ideas in print again, I had a good meeting with the colleagues I was talking about writing a book with, a good lunch with an old friend Matt Barr, and then todays good news. I was in a mood to celebrate as pitiful as I looked. I wanted chocolate, so the next day I dropped by the store to get some. I was determined to enjoy the "up" moments. In a slow moving downward slide of a degenerative disease the up moments—even a steady plateau—can be rare, and needs to be celebrated. Hema stayed over that night. This was probably a mistake, as neither of us slept well. The next night she brought wonderful home cooked food and left for home this time. I missed her but we both got better rest apart. In the middle of the night my mind crept back to the moment she saw me and burst into tears. During the night I was compelled to write down the following lines that were something like what I would like to say to her:

> Don't worry so much, we're gonna be fine
> I can see good things good things, for you and I
> So don't worry so much, smile and be free
> Cause I can see good things, good things, for you and me.
> I believe that there are days of wonder, days of wonder and light, up ahead
> For you and I …

The next day I could see the date window of my watch well enough to see that it has been a day off, probably for some time but—more importantly—well enough to change it.

"Ain't hope grand?!" I emailed to Steve and Art, along with a promise to play music next week. In response, Steve wrote that he had "good heart news" to share as an update on his recent heart scare, and that he has been working on a new verse to the "Prince Phillip" song he was working on. This was a tribute to one of the colorful characters from Forshu in Nova Scotia where Steve and Susan have a house. Phillip now had bladder cancer and is sharing many stories—something which probably gives him hope in his life threatening time. Imagine living in a trailer in Nova Scotia with bladder cancer. As Steve said, he had a million dollar view to experience while essentially dying alone. When people can relate to the information in a way that enables them to share connections to their lives in that moment then it can be a positive dynamic. Yes hope is grand. As Steve said, "Hope *is* grand. I can't imagine life without it." I realized that as grand as hope is, it has to be created, co-created through talk and thoughts and behavior—I was beginning to see the power and importance of what we might call *hopeful communication*.

On Sunday, two days after the injections, I did something I do not think I have ever done, which was to watch both back to back NFL playoff games. I could see the numbers, the faces, and detail that made it such a pleasure. This year I had watched more football than ever. I even watched my old

Clemson Tigers in their lackluster bowl game. Thinking perhaps that this might be the last season I could watch it this well, I resolved to savor and enjoy it as much as possible. What if this season coincided with the end of my ability to watch? I rarely even watch two films back to back but I did make it through the second game (San Francisco and the New York Giants) up until overtime. Throughout the games, Hema called but let me call back during breaks to the games, so I did not miss a moment. I think she knew I was enjoying the experience so much. I wanted to cut a rock again sometime soon. Something I had not done in a while. I wanted to read a book. By the end of game two, my eyes craved to be away from the dazzling, overly hyped, and ever changing televised images of football coverage. They wanted to take the rest of me to bed and peaceful blankness. My eyes led the way assertively.

Hema surprised me on the next rainy Monday morning. She came by on her way to an appointment to bring me a bagel, and to tell me not to walk this day. She made me promise not to go out in the rain as it might get in my eye. I agreed though would probably do so anyway—something she probably also realized! I told her I felt so much better. She was pleased but told me that my eye still looked bad, and to stay in the house today or come over later for food. For the first time in days I was playful with her. I got down on one knee and kissed her hands. I acted like I was getting down in order to kiss her feet, something that she would not let me do, and so on. My Nakuras (theatrics) had returned! She laughed with me, and cautioned me at the same time. She wanted me to come over for dinner, and I said maybe if it is not raining, as driving on dark rainy nights had not changed for the better. This was the morning that Gabby Gifford resigned to focus on recovery. The gist of her resignation statement was that she has the hope of a full recovery over years, not months, but needed to focus on that and not work. It was obvious that she would make a difference for people experiencing similar traumas. How will I make a difference, I thought to myself? Also that morning, on the news, there was the story of a man in Alabama who lost his home and everything in it in a severe storm overnight. His tearful pledge to rebuild, to go on, inspired hope and, again, made me count my blessings and try to be positive about where I was.

Now that I had a major problem of my own, I was beginning to listen to people and empathize with them in ways that I could not before. I drew strength from the resolve of people far worse off than me to move ahead, to rebuild, and to make the most of life. I recognized that I too would not beat the odds on some things. I too was as mortal as everyone else. But I also came to realize that there was hope, which is based on committing energy to speaking, thinking, and making positive things happen. This was the birth of the importance for me of "positive communication" and I decided to teach a course on the subject in the fall of 2012, when I would return from research leave.

Counting Blessings

Counting blessings seemed to be one of the facets of hopeful communication. At about the two week mark, right between the second and upcoming third injection, I got a call one evening around 10pm from an old friend, Tim Biggart. Tim and I had become friends through our common interest in lapidary arts/rock cutting. We used to go to shows to buy rocks, and we had shared a studio downtown for a few years in which we taught people how to do cabochon style stone cutting for jewelry. We kept in touch sporadically after he left Greensboro to teach at Berry College in Georgia. On this night he sounded different. He had just gotten out of hospital for life threatening congestive heart failure. Besides this, he was struggling with diabetes as well as an ear disease that meant he needed strong medication to stop him from experiencing constant vertigo that would otherwise make him fall over. He was unable to drive himself as all of the medications meant he would often fall asleep. He had already banged up the car falling asleep at the wheel on the fifteen minute drive home. He was calling to ask me to come and visit, and cut rocks, go to a rock show in March or June, and generally relive the good times we used to share. His request was punctuated with him telling me how blessed his life is with the following: He loved his wife of thirty-five years more than ever; he was proud of his daughter; he was thankful that he had good friends like me in his life, and so on. He was making a point of letting me know he cared, and that he wanted to see me. I am sure he was shaken deeply by his catastrophic health problems, and by the close call with his own mortality which his hospital stays had made vivid for him. It was good to reconnect and I assured him we would make it out there sometime. He had mentioned dates in March and June. I pledged to myself to try for the March dates not knowing if he would make it to June. We did not make either dates because of family travel plans, but we wanted to. As I told him of my current eye issues, he told me that I was on his prayer list—something I had never heard him talk about before. Could prayer—hopeful communication with God—make a difference? We also shared a moment of lament that stem cell research was not further along. "Just five more years, just five more years", he joked wryly, in fragile hope for future cures for both of us—for me for my sight, and for him for his very life.

Differing Voices and the Beginnings of Self-Empowerment and Advocacy

My doctor had been so happy to share with me the images showing that the edema was going down. He had cautioned me before the first injection that this was not a cure, and that it might not work. So, I knew we were simply trying something that might work here. The drug Avastin was an angiogenesis blocker, designed originally for colorectal cancer treatment. It helped to stop the spread and break up of blood vessels that, in cancer, would feed the tumor, but in the eyes would cause blindness. We hoped that it might just dampen down the swelling and bleeding that was causing the damage to the retina, and related vision loss. So this was very much an "off label" application, even if we might characterize it a little more hopefully than a "Hail-Mary pass" or a "shot in the dark" as it felt to me in darker moments. Dr. Sanders had introduced it to me as a "wonder drug" which had been found to have great possibilities for eye treatment. Thankfully, it seemed to be making a positive difference. I had noticed after a few days that the vision in my right eye was a little clearer. The yellow lines in the road were not bending like spaghetti, if I looked directly at them while driving. Faces on the television were not as distorted or almost blank unless I looked slightly to the left of them. So, I clearly knew and could recollect the voice of medical authority and knowledge at that time which was, "Cause not known" and "No known treatment." This was prominent in the literature as well as face to face meetings with doctors. Unambiguous statements of fact for an academic like me were always suspicious. What were such declaratives designed to smooth over, to obviate, to block from view and from further scrutiny? Just as the blanket statements about people and relationships prevalent in communication textbooks lends themselves to critical reading … "really this is true of relationships everywhere, throughout time and across the broad range of diversity out there?"

I trusted my doctor to do the best he could to help me. I never doubted him. At the same time, my mind would occasionally come back to the odd fact that despite the enormous strides in technology and medical science and research, we currently did not really even know what caused this problem, or what might cure it. Neither was there mention that I could find in the information out there what it might take to make such progress. What type of research would it take? What strides in knowledge are needed to solve this puzzle, or even know what the pieces are? Oddly I could find no visualization of a way forward that is sometimes needed to lead to that way forward. Why were we trying an off-label cure that might help in this day and age, here in the USA? Did we not care about people with vision loss and blindness as much as other diseases and other people? If not, why not? Questions like these pressed on my mind without answers.

Three days later on the following Monday, I notice on Facebook the complaints about the gloom and drizzle of the Monday morning. Perhaps people are partly complaining about going back to work, but I remember being so thankful for a gloomy day. It is ironic that I had always enjoyed, and being drawn to, sunny weather. My mind flashed back to some of the times I complained about the gloomy British weather when I was home for summer holidays. I felt guilty now that I had complained so many times about the weather, over which my family had no control. Now, I could see so much better on that overcast day as I walked around the nearby upper middle class neighborhood with my neighbor friend John. I was not battling to avoid the bright sun. He talked about his legal woes in dealing with the fallout of his failed marriage to a Russian woman he had sponsored contractually to come to the US. I counted my blessings—at least I had a great partner who vowed to stay with me. I was not a "cash cow" for someone who wishes me just enough harm that I am miserable, but not quite so much that I cannot provide ongoing and consistent funds for them. This seemed to be John's situation, at least as he narrated it. His contractual deal with her would likely be until death, but he too was struggling and battling away in his own story, as was I. In an unspoken way, as we walked, we shared this common sense of battling something malevolent in our respective lives.

On that particular walk, I knew my eye was an awful sight and I was in the middle of a bad cold I seemed to catch as soon as I walked out of the doctor's office. The slight choking feeling had gone, and I was up for a good roam around the area neighborhoods, and some fresh air and conversation. He listened to my woes, and I could tell he was processing the information. A day or two later, during the president's state of the Union Address one evening, I got a series of texts from him. They clustered around the idea that he thinks my doctor is trying to mask the underlying problem, and that the injections may hurt me more than help. He went on to tell me that I needed to become "the expert" and to look for the origin of the problem. He went on to tell me that the AMA exists not to cure people, but to make money, and that if I understood this I was already beginning to take control.

I responded with a thanks, and that there is not much information out there that sheds light on its origins, other than to designate it a genetic mutation that may or may not be inherited. He then recounted a tale of a man he met who was suicidal from chronic headaches that baffled even the people at the Mayo Clinic. He visited a Chinese acupuncturist who found him allergic to sulphites and, upon eliminating them from his diet, was almost instantly cured. I did not respond, but I tried respectfully to take in his perspective. Such cases do exist, and perhaps there was an alternative way to discover the core underlying issue. At the same time I was left uneasy by this new ambiguity. Perhaps I was approaching this all wrong. Perhaps I was missing something that others understood clearly, and achieved the cure they were looking for? Do I have a problem that is curable or not? Who can tell me for sure? Certainly the traditional medical model voice was very clear—we will try something that *might* work but, otherwise, we do not really know cause or cure. Would seeking alternatives be a wild goose chase to nowhere, or was there a magic cure out there that a paradigm shift in how we approach medicine might reveal? Was I simply being caught betwixt and between discourses that did not mix well, or was it really worth exploring? If so, where and how should I begin? Again, I had no idea.

So at that point, a few days after the second injections, I was left with some very definite and unambiguous statements from the medical world (this is the way it is and were doing what we can—follow the prescribed course of treatment), which gave rise to some shaky but nagging questions and doubts in the back of my head (why is it the way it is, and how can I be smart about what is happening?). I had John's perspective which was bordering on conspiratorial (do not believe them or accept that this is the way it is. Take charge of your experience–be a smart consumer) Coupled with this was the caring and accommodating voices I was hearing from my dean and department head at my workplace, where I would be back to full-time teaching in just a few months (we will purchase what equipment you might need, let us know). Additionally I was hearing loving and caring voices from family and my partner ("I will be your eyes, my love" as Hema said several times). I was hearing caring reassurances from the world around me, but at the same time I was still struck with the deeper questions of why this disease, and why me? All of the help started to sound like it was organized around me losing my sight—we will help you cope with the inevitable. Others had resolved themselves to my truth much quicker than I had. Better to have those caring voices, certainly, but it was an oddly double-sided comfort for me. At least that is how I heard things at the time.

I spent some time sorting through these voices and resolved to make the most of, and be grateful for, their caring messages. Taking the best of each, I resolved to build relationships with people I could talk to about this and rely on as caring friends; to research more on alternative health possibilities and be as smart as I could be whatever that meant; be smart and informed about what I needed to live and work as well as I could; and to also accept the expertise of my medical crew who, I believed, were helping not hurting me.

During the four weeks after the second injection, I had a constant wheeze and cold. I refused to take medications for symptoms of the Avastin—thinking that was another slippery slope I needed to avoid. It seemed, at least from television ads for medications, that the pharmaceutical industry gained much from people taking medications by offering to treat the symptoms, and side effects of their medication. The side effects often appeared worse than the original diseases, at least to someone who did not have those diseases. Instead, I resolved to work out, eat healthily, minimize the place of chemicals and toxins from packaged foods and other sources in my life, and stay as positive as possible. I researched sunglasses that would make walking in the sun less painful, and I cut the first stone I had cut in a long time. I cut a piece of Petoskey stone Art had given me. It was something he had since his childhood days. I cut it for him and gave it back to him so he could enjoy seeing it in this polished and symmetrical form. I think he was assuming I would keep it, but I wanted him to have it.

Not long before my third injection, my old pal Bud Goodall checked in with me on Facebook after I asked him about his return to chemo for his pancreatic cancer. I updated him on my situation. The interaction ended:

"I will pray for you my friend" he said.

"And I will pray for you" I replied.

"We always did make a good team" he said.

"Yes, we did, and we're still in the game …" he had logged out as I wrote this last comment. His encouraging and empathic voice was so important to me during this time.

· 5 ·

THIRD INJECTION

February 17th 2012

The second injection made a difference in terms of improving my vision but not as much as the first injection. Perhaps the Avastin was also holding off any new developments. If so, that was something good on top of the improvements it had made. I was a little surprised when Matt the technician told me that the right eye had improved since the last time four weeks ago because the letter tests always seemed like a struggle and a disappointment for me. I could not articulate how my sight had improved but it had, so things remained on a positive note. I did ask him this time how my eyes faired compared to the driving test requirements. He simply said, "they're about there" at the 20/40 level necessary, although he just told me I was at a 20/60 level! I was a little confused, but left this topic alone as I did not want to raise any flags. Getting around would be so difficult if I had to stop driving, and I did not know what the information sharing between clinic and DMV consisted of, if any. A friend had recently had her license suspended for a while because of a seizure, so I know offices can talk. I wanted to keep driving as long as I could and see how this course of treatment played out. Perhaps it would bump me into an acceptable level of acuity. That was the best possible scenario anyway. I felt that I could still see well enough close to home where I knew the roads, lights, and signs. After the obligatory retinal pictures, I moved quickly through to the consulting room where Dr. Sanders would meet with me to do the injections, and to touch base on how things looked at this point.

He came in and was upbeat and positive like last time. He showed me the pictures of my retinas on the monitor screen, and told me that the swelling had gone down. He was resolute again in wanting us to see the four injections through as a course of treatment. I agreed. He said that there should be no reason why, at some point soon, I would no longer need more of the injections, though it was hard for me to imagine at this point. He assured me that, even though I was an anomaly in terms of having the bulls eye maculopathy as a relatively young man, I could expect to return to just having that problem and not the additional swelling and bleeding. I would never have "normal" vision again, but to beat this complication would be a significant victory for us. His confidence in the treatment process was comforting.

"So it's possible that the treatment could actually stop the retina complications?" I asked for clarification.

"Not only is it possible, I would say it's very probable. Yes!" He replied confidently and reassuringly.

I wanted so much to believe him. I really wanted what he was saying to come true—as much for Hema as for myself. I knew she so much wanted me to be alright for our life together. He then decided to look through the microscope. He dictated some notes to the heavily pregnant Amanda as he did so. He then backed off his optimism just slightly. He said that a small area of new bleeding had emerged in the right eye, and that there was a tiny cyst in the left eye that we would look closely at next time. He asked me if I had noticed any problems with vision in the left eye. I said that it sometimes took a few seconds for the left eye to "sort of warm up and get into focus." He told the technician that we would do an angiogram next time. "I want to get the total picture of the landscape that we're looking at" he said. "Ok, that sounds good" I replied.

He looked slightly troubled by the last part of what he saw. Again, I was left with a tantalizing cliff-hanger somewhere around cautionary good news but with no clear sense of an overall definitive account of what was happening. Perhaps this narrative space is good. At least it provided for hope as well as the darker nervousness and fear. I was right on the edge of a happy and an unhappy story and we did not know yet how the landscape would unfold. I could tell from his ordering of tests that would provide him with the "total landscape" that he was also craving a narrative that plausibly connected the dots, and captured what was happening. Where would the story go from here? This was too much of a mystery for both of us, although it is a narrative moment everyone faces in their life in their own way, often many times. At the same time not having narrative closure meant that we would keep trying, there was room for hope. As Bud would later say, "no bad news is good news."

I noted to myself that he was mentioning cysts for the first time. What did that mean, and how was it related to the edema he talked about last time? I asked him what this meant, and he explained that tiny fluid sacks were forming and impacting the retina. But still, neither of us had anything like a complete sense of the dynamics of what was happening. The all-important "why?" was still missing for us, and we did not know when it would emerge, if ever. But we would know more next time and, perhaps, it would all come together clearly at the end of the fourth injection. I was being urged to stay tuned to my own story, and it felt surreal, odd, fearful, and dangerous.

As he was preparing to put the numbing needle into my eye, he asked me how my last name was pronounced. Were the t's silent, something like Kellee? I told him the correct pronunciation. He always tried to take my mind off the incoming needles just before the injections. After the injection, I told him there were more people with that name in the upstate of SC where I used to live.

"You mean around Greenville?"

"Yes and Seneca where I lived for a few years" I replied.

"I went to Clemson" he said, surprised by our common history. We had talked about this before but it was a while ago and, understandably, he seemed to have forgotten.

We connected briefly on our mutual experience of that place again. We also successfully positioned the injection into a conversation about something else, which was comforting. He asked me what I taught there and I told him "Communication"

"Oh, I wish we would have had a course in that in med. school" he said.

"I know some programs are now integrating communication into med school curricula" I replied.

"Doctor—patient communication is important I know." I added.

"Oh yes" he said.

"You're very good at it!" I said.

"Well thanks! That means a lot, especially coming from a professional. Ok I'll see you next time" he concluded.

He was off to the next waiting patient. I made an appointment for four weeks, and was out into the bright light once again to drive cautiously home on my preplanned and familiar route.

I rested that day. As I did so, I searched for an image—perhaps a metaphor—to capture where we were with this treatment. I know it felt like living in an eternal cliff-hanger of not having the closure or clarity of an explanation. As such, it felt a little blunt—crude—something to try that might just do the trick. Maybe it was like spray hosing an area where brush fires were popping up. Not knowing why the fires were occurring or if and when new fires would pop up. We simply resolved to keep "hosing" the retinas down with medication in hopes that the fires would go out. A cruder image might be that we were shooting something until whatever it was that was attacking me simply stopped moving. Something was still struggling to move—to express itself almost like a living entity—I could almost feel it. I had an intuition that a new area was becoming a problem in the right eye, which turned out to be true. Perhaps something was also stirring in the left eye. With these metaphoric images, I was trying my best to avoid the "battle" metaphor that, to me, seemed a little patronizing, although perhaps some were inspired by it. Yet, it was taking on somewhat the form of a battle. A largely unknown enemy was attacking me for reasons that were unclear, and we were counter-attacking it with the sustained methodical use of the one weapon we were sure we had—Avastin. How smart, persistent, and resourceful the enemy was against a one pronged defense we did not really know yet. Neither did I know what other defenses, if any, I might be able to add to our repertoire of weapons and tactics.

Hema came over in the evening to take care of me. She had made my favorite Sāmbhar and rice with a side of potatoes and kale. Simple and delicious! As she walked in she told me I looked a lot better than last time. I fe lt right away also that the side effects had not hit me as hard this time. Perhaps last time some of it got back behind my throat and sinuses. It felt quite a bit different this time, although I was careful to avoid crowds given the weakness of my immune system after the last injection.

That evening after dinner we watched Wall St 2. Gordon Geko was back from the 1980s to define unfounded speculation as the root of all evil. Perhaps this was true in the Wall Street crash to which his character was referring, but smart speculative guess work was what we were going with for my treatment. It was the only hope we had. The movie was a nice distraction from the discomfort of my treatment, and a great performance by Michael Douglas, but I gave up with forty-five minutes to go. My eyes just were too tired from the battering of the day to follow the many twists and turns of the story towards the end of the film. Hema would recount and complete the rest of the story for me the next morning, and the twists and turns of the story were many and surprising. I could relate.

To Share or Not to Share: Learning to Express

By this point in February 2012, there were several people who were familiar with the routine of treatment I was on, and who would check in for updates on the story after each injection. This engagement of others in my story was a very meaningful way of sharing the stress and, at the same time, making sense of it for me. It also enabled them to connect to my experience, and show that they cared. I edited and emphasized slightly different things as I reported the updates to different people. For dad, I shared what happened during the treatment, what we now know, and what would come next—procedural facts. Mum connected more on the side effects given that she had suffered from the side effects and interactions of medications for many years. Several friends just wanted me to know they were keeping track of the dates and main events. Some friends simply asked periodically how my eyes were doing and left it open-ended for me to share what I wanted to share. By mid-February even Hema's mother was asking for updates on how I was doing—her way of communicating through Hema that she liked me, and cared about me. Although we had not yet met, she made sure Hema fed me well before and after injections on the assumption that good food was important when taking medications. We had recently received a package of her home made Sāmbhar powder which was exceptionally good. She and Hema's dad and sisters included a really nice Shaffer pen as a gift for me. I was looking forward to meeting my Indian family someday soon and seeing their lives first hand—and sharing some of our life with them.

By the third week of February it felt like spring was in the air. On February 21st I spent a good hour pruning and feeding the roses and fruit trees. I got caught up with the compost production for this year. I spent some time digging in the leaves I had shredded in the fall so that the vegetable patch would be moving towards preparation for planting. The normality of these early spring chores felt so good. Of course we could still get a wintry blast or two but I noticed the fruit tree branches I pruned were green with life, and the nectarine trees were actually on the verge of flowering. I hoped it was not too soon for them. That afternoon I got a card from one of my gym buddies—Kate—saying that the gym was not the same without me, and that I was missed. I was really touched to know that I was not forgotten. Now that the days were getting longer I would be back soon, as driving there in the early morning would not be so scary for me. I cooked for Hema and, I recall, that at 6:15 pm when she arrived, there was still some light in the dusky sky. With the spring came light and green life and, for me, an easier time to drive in the mornings and at night.

By this time in February we were more open to sharing my condition with people, and I was becoming more comfortable with people knowing this most personal of issues. I am a private person, so this was not easy for me. However, sharing information was especially useful when it helped avoid misunderstandings and resulting miscommunication. There were a couple of times, for example, when I did not recognize someone because their face appeared blank. Naturally they seemed puzzled that I was not responding to them. Clarifying that I was not ignoring them, but that my eye condition means that sometimes I do not recognize faces, helped avoid awkward miscommunication. I became proactive, and matter of fact, in clarifying things like this when these situations arose.

Sharing details of my condition and related experiences was also valuable in building connections with people who knew much more than I did about vision loss and blindness. I made an appointment with Bill, our new graduate school Dean, for me and Kolby to meet with him. He has a strong background in working with blind people and researching blindness. I met Kolby and Sunny outside the EUC and she took my arm as we walked over to Bills office. As we walked, she asked me all about how my vision was, and how I was coping. Bill was gracious enough to meet with us for an hour even though he was pushed for time between meetings. We all talked, and he and Kolby found many connections in common. As they talked, I found myself thinking to myself that I did not want to be one of the people they were talking about. I admired Kolby enormously, but at this point I could not imagine living her life. It would be such an enormous existential and practical change. As I sat with them in Bills office, I realized I had started to open up to people who could, and would, help me. Afterwards, I walked Kolby back to her dorm and we resolved to get together again soon. "Keep in touch," she texted me later. Of course I would!

In March, the weather was so Spring-like that I committed to spending at least an hour per day, weather permitting, to yard work. This could be the spring that I really get on top of yard projects, as I have the time and the physical/outdoor hour is a nice break from writing. I cleared out the weeds from the fruit beds, pruned, trimmed, and dug out the one or two trees that did not make it from what I planted last year. It was good to be out in the yard where things were starting to bloom and come back to life. The nectarines were blooming and they were, to use an old saying with new meaning, "a sight for sore eyes"! I had begun to make sure I enjoyed what I saw of nature, and of the world immediately around me that I had had a hand in shaping. To see a bird land in a tree that I had planted last year or the year before, to see irises come up that I had planted three or four years ago, and to see the dirt of my vegetable patch crumble as I walked on it—a sign of its huge progress from thick clay when I bought the house—were rich and good moments. I was a small man who had made a small difference to a small place in a corner of the world, and I enjoyed savoring all of the signs of this. In the beauty of springtime my mind focused a lot more on the bright side of all of this, rather than the darker possibilities of this being among the last years I might see all of this as well as I did now. Something about spring brought green living hope to life. I cleared out an entire chest of drawers for Hema to put her things in so that she had enough clothes to stay for a whole weekend if she wanted to. I also vowed for March to stop my nightly glass of wine, no chocolate or any other pre-packaged junk, and to seriously kick start the process of getting back in shape and purifying what goes into my body. It had to make a difference somehow, and this seemed like a good place and time to start.

The day after Valentine's-day my cat died. She had been suffering from kidney failure for over a year. She crawled onto me one last time as I watched the BBC news that morning. Then, as I began writing, she squawked to go out. It was a very assertive squawk. I checked on her after a while and saw that she was on her favorite chair on the front porch, curled up and sleeping. It was the last time I saw her. The next time I checked she had wandered off to die. I wondered if she had a spot picked out, or if she had simply walked until she found somewhere to hide and curl up one last time. A week or two later I emailed several people who had known her well to let them know. I contacted Alex who knew her while we were dating around ten years earlier. We exchanged news, she was dating a new woman in New York; real-estate sales were slow in Boston, and so on. I did not share information about my eyes. Why would she or any exes want to know about that? I wondered momentarily how many exes would be relieved that they did not get stuck with someone who was losing their sight. It was a moment of self- pity I am guessing that many in my position would experience. I told her about Hema. We were both pleased for each other. We kept things light and breezy and got caught up on personal/relational news instead.

There are some situations where it is just best not to share ones problems. Sharing one's story has its boundaries. During a hair-cut, my stylist found it funny that I had missed a spot on the far left of my face while shaving, and that I had hacked my left sideburn in an attempt to trim it a few days earlier. Why burden everyone with the heaviness of a problem when there is nothing they can do, and probably do not need to know? Awkwardness is so awkward! After all, as Bud told me years ago, what is at the center of your world is not necessarily, and often is not, at the center of other peoples' worlds. Why suck them across the line into your dark side when they were having a perfectly happy day cutting hair or doing whatever they did, and having a laugh at your clumsiness?

What to share and what not to share were important decisions in close relationships also. In fact, constructing this imaginary line between what is shared and not is something I would have to become smarter at, and more sensitive to. How to share was as important as what to share. Mid-March was Hema's spring break and she stayed with me most of the week. During that time we talked more about when we would live together permanently. As part of that discussion we talked about where we would live. She wanted to move to a bigger house where we would have more personal space. She did not want to move into my current house, and then have to move again in a year or two. That would be complicated, and she was right—I understood. I think she had a good point on several levels. More space would be good. Somewhere new would make it more special and avoid issues relating to moving into my established territory. At the same time I was reluctant to start a new mortgage, and move, unless we could do a fifteen year mortgage, and if we could live within walking distance to a good grocery store. I was conscious of my need to be close to a food source without driving for times when Hema was not around. If I had to give up driving, and Hema was out of town, then I needed to be able to take care of myself. She agreed, and we narrowed our parameters to integrate both of our desires. We were negotiating, and we would come back to this later to refine our desires to meet both our needs as, to her, I just sounded pessimistic instead of cautious.

She asked me as we were driving along one day, what kind of car I would want next. I hesitated to respond but told her that I was happy with my current car. Although it was twelve years old at the time, it was still a good car and I did not see the need to change it. I also said that I did not know if I would ever need another car, as I did not know how long I would be driving for. Perhaps I did not need to share this fear. It was not what she wanted to hear. She told me to be positive, and that she knew I would be driving for at least another twenty years. I knew this was highly unlikely, but stayed quiet—not wanting to sound pessimistic again. A few days earlier I had looked at my driver's license, and noted that it expired in 2015. For me this meant that I would have to retake the eye test at that point to get it renewed—a test I feared even now, three years from the expiration date. If I failed the test, I thought to myself, I would be done with driving, so why buy a new car before then? I chose not to share this thought with Hema because it just would not have helped anything during her Spring break. I wanted her to rest and relax a bit, and adding my worries to the conversation would not have helped. I let the car discussion fade away into the backdrop of errands and activities that made up her week off.

Maybe it was the spring, and maybe partly the discussion of new houses and the future generally, the topic of whether we would have a baby came up. It was a multilayered issue for me, and I am not sure how I reacted when Hema would bring this up. I think I just went quiet. I know she wanted a child. She would be a wonderful mother. At the same time I was about to turn fifty. I did not know if I would be disabled in the next year or two. If so, would I be able to provide for them? Could Hema take care of both of us? When, if ever, would I be able to retire, if I was able to go on working? Would it not be better to plan to be able to retire as soon as possible if I was having major problems seeing? As is true many times in life there is always the crossroads moment between taking the risk that things will be alright, and not taking the risk and wishing you did, looking back later. The crossroads nature of this decision was no more vivid than in the fact that if my disease was genetic in origin, then I had a 50/50 chance of passing it on to our child if we had one. Once again, I needed to get better at engaging with these conversations rather than just sort of freezing and not knowing what to say, or just letting Hema do most of the talking until the topic drained away. She would notice at some point soon that I was not contributing much to the discussion but, much of the time, I just did not know what to say.

Some unusual aspects of the experience are just not easily communicable. I am not sure exactly when it began but there were times when I would close my eyes at the end of the day and see a light feature, like a cloud, with a brighter feature within it. It looked like an image of the universe with the inner area consisting of more densely spaced stars and the outer ones where the stars spanned out into the nothingness of space. As I tried to focus on the inner bright area, it would morph and change as if I had an image of part of the universe at the back of my eye. I do not know if this is what they mean by "floaters" but it was an odd phenomenon. It reduced when my right eye started to respond positively to treatment, so perhaps my eyes were picking up and processing an image of the swelling activity in the eye. There were times also when beautiful abstract patterns with unnamable colors would appear before my closed eyes. I wished I could have captured them in some art form, like painting. It was a physically pleasurable feeling to see the images, but I had no way to capture in words or communicate what they were like. I wished I could have. They were really beautiful and other-worldly.

Managing the line between expressing and not expressing difficult emotions, like anger and frustration, would be one that I continued to find difficult. Mostly I experienced anger and frustration at my own struggles with technology. For example, we had begun the important tasks of looking into the flights and hotel accommodations for the trip we had planned to visit my family in England that summer. I remember looking at a web page for a hotel near my parent's house, and trying to find out how much it would cost for the stay we had planned. The page kept defaulting back to June dates even though I was searching for information about July. I got so angry when it wouldn't work for me I shouted, "Fuck it. Fuck it!" I stormed away from the computer.

"What's wrong?" Hema asked, shocked and upset by my outburst.

"It won't fucking work for me. It keeps changing the dates I type in"

"It's ok, it's ok!" she tried to calm me.

"It's not ok. I can't see the damn thing properly" I maintained my angry performance.

"I understand" she said.

"You don't understand. You don't understand," I replied, storming into the bedroom. I felt like I was turning into a bloody drama queen, but I could not help it!

She went onto the website and clicked on the keys for a minute. I had apparently forgotten that the day and month are reversed in England. I had been typing in a date expecting to see their cost for dates which had already passed for this year! That's why the site kept defaulting to another date. I would have to get better at channeling and expressing my emotions, or I would continue to drag Hema into my needless theatrics, which always stressed her out, reminding her of her father, and her first marriage.

The early spring was a wonderful time, being so full of life and love and plans for the summer and beyond. At the same time there were private moments I did not share with anyone, where I would simply feel intense disappointment. Not really anger, not really frustration or fear, just deep, deep cavernous disappointment. This was supposed to be the time ahead for so much to happen, so many good things to enjoy, and I did not know where it was all going. I felt the story I desired slipping away from me, and I had no control over it.

· 6 ·

FOURTH INJECTION

March 20th 2012

Despite the existentially heavy moments of disappointment, overall I was feeling quite good going into the fourth injection. I did not notice any deterioration in my eye sight although, as the appointment drew nearer, I was reminded of Dr. Sander's slight worry last time. I knew I would have a battery of tests before the fourth injection and it would be a crucial visit. It would also be a crucial month to follow, in deciding what I needed from this point forward.

As the late spring grew brighter in mid-March, and the days grew longer, I began to think about buying a better pair of sunglasses. This may seem trivial to someone who does not have this disease, but it has a way of shifting perceptions and priorities in odd and surprising ways. This was the only marked adjustment I felt like I needed at this point, besides sometimes sitting close to the television to minimize distortion of images. I currently had several pairs of sunglasses, but they all dated back to times when I was not experiencing sensitivity to sunlight as I now did. I never paid more than about $20 for a pair as they often got lost, scratched, or sat on by me. For walks now I needed some that were much better at cutting the harsh glare of the sun than the regular sunglasses I had picked up here and there. Also, I did not want light getting in over the tops of my glasses, and none of the pairs I currently had worked well enough to meet both needs. The glasses I liked were around $200, so it was not an easy decision given that they rarely lasted long for me. I held off making a purchase, thinking that the fourth injection visit might provide more clarity on what I needed.

It was just before the 4th injection that I began in earnest to look online for clues as to the origins and preventative steps advised for people with wet macular degeneration. Why I left this research so late I do not know. Perhaps I was realizing that it would not be something that we simply zapped with the Avastin and moved on. Perhaps my mind was focused more on the primary disease I had been dealing with—the Cone Dystrophy, and I saw the macular degeneration as a "complication" of that. In reality, the macular degeneration was a much bigger and more immediate threat, but we just had not named it as such until now. I realized at this point that I had two major diseases attacking my eyes at the same time—so every day that I could do normal tasks relatively easily seemed like a genuine blessing to me. This was going to be a struggle, and perhaps some other lifestyle changes might make a difference. I had looked at a few sources early on for information on the Cone Dystrophy, but now I was curious about the macular disease to which the Cone Dystrophy seemed to have made me predisposed. I wanted to understand more about why I might have been predisposed to the macular disease. I was something of an anomaly in developing this so early in life, and was curious about why. I also wanted to explore strategies beyond the injections that might help. There had to be things I could do in addition to, and between, the monthly injections that might help to at least slow the disease, and I knew that I would have to explore these strategies for myself.

Discussing nutrition, lifestyle choices, and so on, were never part of the focused and quick treatment discussions with my ophthalmologist, but that did not mean they were unimportant. In fact, these were discussions that I would have with Hema on an ongoing basis. The information I found, mostly online, would become important in framing certain aspects of how we lived. I had no idea if adapting to preventative steps for something that might be genetic, or caused by the Cone Dystrophy, would make a difference. But it was something to try, that just might make a difference. So I began exploring websites and online sources related to preventative steps that might impact macular degeneration. Hema and I would discuss these, and we made some efforts to adjust diet and lifestyle to accommodate the online wisdom we found.

Dreams, Metaphors, and Reality

A couple of nights before the fourth injection I had a dream in which I walked into class on the first day of the fall. In the dream, I told my students that I needed them to say my name when they wanted my attention, as I would find it difficult to see their hands go up in the air when they wanted to speak. Someone told me that I needed a certain official colored dot—red I think it was—on the syllabus to be classified as "visually impaired." I did not have the dot, so some of them expressed concern that I was not officially impaired. I think some actually walked out of the classroom because I did not have the correct dot. Bureaucracy never sleeps! Was I worried about being a fraud? Was I worried about the reaction of students as I might begin to need to tell them up front? It was certainly an odd dream that abruptly woke me. Was I wondering about where I was on the scale between normal and impaired—how much sight have I currently lost? Probably, yes. Was I worried about how my sight would be by August, and how it would affect teaching—would I be officially "visually-impaired" by then, whatever that meant? Probably, that was also true. Was I worried about what would transpire at the next appointment? Definitely! I was nervous about this pivotal moment, as it would decide if treatment had been successful or if I needed more injections and, if so, how often. There was always the nagging possibility—actually I thought it was more of a probability—that this same problem could also start occurring in the left eye; the one I thought was going to carry me through more or less ok. Having one "good eye" was a constant relief, but how long this would last was a low humming and ever present worry for me. We simply did not know, and I had already been perilously close to needing treatment in it.

On this visit, I had a new nurse to walk me through the eye tests and retinal photographs needed for Dr. Sanders to evaluate where I was, and what we would need from here. They always began with questioning what, if any, changes I had noticed. I thought things were about the same, but certainly no better. She told me I did just one letter better on the reading test, which backed up my perceptions that there was no significant changes in either direction. I asked her what might be the bright luminescent gray cloud-like image I often saw when I closed my eyes. She told me it was probably the area of the eye being treated. Somehow my eye was seeing an image of the area of my retina in which the Avastin was working. There were many such surreal moments and experiences over the months. She took my eye pressure, dilated my eyes, and we were off to the photography room.

She took some pictures, but needed my eyes to be more dilated so we waited a few minutes. I curled my toes to help the dilation—a trick I had been taught on a previous visit. While waiting, I asked her how, in her experience, the technology we were sitting among had changed the work they do. Interestingly, she remembered the time around the year 2000, just before digital technology had made diagnostics so thorough and instant. Back then, the pictures would be taken much as they are now but then the negatives were either processed in a dark room on the premises, or they would be sent out for processing. The patient would wait for a few days and then come back when the photographs were processed—much like the way holiday/vacation pictures were done before the digital age. Of course the images then were flat two dimensional pictures and, as she put it, "largely just to document things." What did she mean by "just documenting things" I asked? She went on to tell me that before the Avastin was applied to the treatment of wet macular degeneration (in 2005) and since then other drugs, they were largely just documenting the progress of the disease as there was nothing they could do to stop it. Just a few years after Avastin came to be the "go to" drug for wet macular degeneration, the company producing it tried to replace it with another product specifically for eyes, but which did essentially the same thing as Avastin. Avastin costs $85 per shot, which we do once a month. The other drug (Lucentis) costs over $2000 per shot. So you can see why the company was keen to replace it! A now legendary battle ensued between the company and outraged Ophthalmologists, led by Dr. Rosenthal at Bascom Palmer (who I would later meet in person). The doctors managed to maintain the accessibility of Avastin to the thousands of people in the US and around the world who probably could not afford the expensive replacement. It would have been tough (but possible) for me to spend $2000 plus per month for treatment, but impossible for many—especially those without insurance. I felt both fortunate at that moment, and sad for others who did not have access to what I had. At least I had a chance. Yes, I knew that a few years from now there would be new technologies and drugs—advances I wished for now—but just a few years ago people would have dreamed of the treatment possibilities I had, as basic, blunt, and uncertain as they now seemed to be to me. Treatment is a "progressive" discourse like other discourses in which we are always hoping for a better approach ahead, and in which those gone before us never quite had what we had. The conflict over Avastin also tells us that the "progress" is rarely smooth or politically and economically uncomplicated, but is, itself marked by struggle—most vividly by the apparently competing interests of accessibility/availability and profit.

She took multiple pictures of both eyes, both before and after injecting dye into my bloodstream. The dye made me extremely nauseas for a few seconds. She moved a trash can close to me in case I was sick, but it passed quickly, and I was fine. The world was a surreal and beautiful bright pink to me as I walked out into the waiting room, and on to a consulting room to meet with Dr. Sanders.

Dr. Sanders started the consultation by asking me how things had gone this month. I told him I thought things were about the same, which he affirmed with a glance at the eye test results. We looked through images of the right eye, and he told me that we would have to continue monthly treatments as the bleeding was still active. We were both disappointed, but at least it looked like the Avastin was holding off any significant worsening. We then turned to the pictures of the left eye and looked through many images together. He also looked through the microscope into the eye. He told me that at some point we might have to start treating the left eye with injections. Again, we were both disappointed that our ideal storyline was being replaced by one that was grounded in resolute but cautious optimism. He could see a small area of bleeding developing in that eye also. This was just what we did not want. Although he was heartened by the fact that the profile images of the retina showed no swelling yet, which explains the relatively good sight in the left eye I still had. The conversational moment was intense but it moved too quickly between images and talk, and back again to images, for a sense of dark foreboding to really take hold for me. I only remember the following talk:

"Can you see the coral reef like structure over here in the right eye?" He asked.

"Yes" I replied.

"Then off over here the new spots of bleeding?" He added.

"Yes" I replied again.

"And here in the left eye there's a small are of bleeding starting" He said.

"Uggh, yes I see that" I replied, unable to ignore the big picture emerging. Things were still perilously active, and now in both eyes.

While he was pointing these things out to me I was thinking, I have something like a barrier structure made of blood vessels building in my eye. As this continues to form, perhaps now in both eyes, I can only imagine the difficulty ahead of trying to see through and around something like a coral reef!

So what we were hoping might have been the final treatment at least for a while was now looking more like just the fourth injection in a series, the length of which was as yet to be determined, and which might involve both eyes. He gave me the injection as I stared at Lauren's sweet index finger to distract me from the incoming needle. Momentarily I imagined Lauren holding up her middle finger instead just for a change—something that, of course, she would never do. The private and fleeting image of absurdity helped me through the moment where the needle came towards my eye. This was the worst moment, knowing that it is coming at you Lauren then carefully washed my eye. The cool cleaning liquid poured painlessly over my eye ball as my lid flapped around, but I knew the battle was just heating up. He told me that we would continue with monthly injections—the "most aggressive" we could be, he emphasized. We were definitely at a crossroads, but it would still take a while to know which way things would go. The answer to the question of where this was all going was always fleetingly, flirtingly, frustratingly, beyond our little grasping finger tips.

I had become tuned into the nuances of verbal and nonverbal cues that Dr. Sanders communicated. He had gone from cautiously optimistic to somewhere between encouragingly neutral and worriedly hopeful. Was this the turning point before more difficult times ahead, or a prelude to stability? Of course we did not know, but the question kept insisting itself into things, like a steely needle. His final words, "Hang in there, and if you notice any major changes, let me know. Don't wait for your next appointment." The words were different from our usual optimistic parting ritual, and hung heavily with me as I made my next appointment at the front desk.

The Reason We Came into Each Other's' Lives

I stepped out into the blinding bright light and drove home, wishing for some cloud-cover but thankful that the roads were quiet. I made it home without any problems. I was thankful to get into the darkened house. I ate some of the leftover food that Hema had cooked for us, and went to bed to rest my eyes. Two hours later, when I awoke, my eyes were no longer heavily dilated but the right eye was very sore. I could barely open it. I had explained this part to people as feeling like I had been punched in the eye, and it did. The left one was also tired from the battering of flash pictures and stinging drops. I lay there, going back over the appointment and the meeting with Dr. Sanders in my mind. As I did, I was filled with fear and sadness, and that looming feeling of disappointment I had felt before. Somewhere in the neighborhood I heard the tuneful sound of an ice cream van, and my mind slipped back to the simple joys of childhood that this sound evoked—a time when small things like running to the van for an ice cream were an urgent wonder, and when sorrows only lasted for a moment, and scrapes quickly healed.

I came quickly back to the fearfulness of where I was in my life now. Would I be able to provide for Hema? Would I be able to take her to some of the places she dreamed of? Would I be able to help make some of her dreams come true in this lifetime, as well as some of my own? Everything seemed to be in question, and in doubt. I tried to hold at bay feelings of unfairness because, honestly, I had had a good life that was better than the lives that many people lived. I rested for the afternoon, as these dark thoughts waned a little. Listening to the news, it was the day that Mitt Romney became "the etch-a-sketch candidate"—a minor news day and an image that only popped up occasionally in the presidential race to follow. I waited limply for the stinging eye pain to subside, and for Hema to come over after work.

Hema called on the way over to ask if I needed anything from the store. I told her we did not need anything for dinner, or for tonight. I could tell she wanted to go to the store to get me something—probably a treat of some kind—but I insisted on her not spending anything. We did not need anything. She came to my house right from work and barely got in the door before she was cooking for us. I do not think she even changed out of the dress shoes she wore for teaching all day. I looked at her adoringly, but she was busy cooking. What she was able to do with some chick peas, spices, and vegetables was amazing. I mostly stayed out of the kitchen when the cooking began in order to avoid the spicy wafting of the cooking pot and, at her request, I relaxed while she did everything.

Yesterday, or the day before—I could not remember which, there was a big crashing thud coming from the kitchen, from near the garden window was my guess. It was so sudden and loud I was afraid to see what it was in case someone was breaking in, or if something had collapsed. After a minute or two I went into the kitchen to see what had happened and there was nothing out of place. Tonight as I took the scraps from Hema's cooking preparations out to the compost bins, seeing something just under the garden window which stuck out from the house, it all suddenly made sense. There, lay a medium sized bird, now dead and buzzing with flies. The poor thing had flown right into the garden window and died then or soon after. It must have lost its way or could not see that it was going right towards an immoveable and deadly window. I did not want to over interpret this or other coincidences as symbolism for my life, but it was certainly poignant on a day like today. It struck me that it does not take much to bring a body to helplessness or demise. The macula is a tiny part of the body, and yet it can change everything so devastatingly quickly, as my window had done for this poor little bird.

The food was wonderful. As we ate on trays on the couch she asked me, "What would you do if I wasn't in your life?"

"I'm not sure" I replied. "Probably go on as best I could for a while until I can't see and then I don't know. I dunno, maybe people back in the old days would just take some pills and be done with it. What would they have done? At least now there's something we can try" I added. Hema listened and waited for me to continue.

"I guess in India there's always someone who will take you in if you're blind?" I asked, using the word blind for the first time today.

"Yes probably. Unless you really pissed off everyone in your family, someone would take you in" she replied.

"I guess that's one upside of a collectivist culture. Are there homes for blind people here in the US, like charity places they would have in the UK? I don't really know. But I can't imagine going back home. This is my home, but I am not sure what I would do." I replied, the missing and unspoken part of this sentence clearly being, "… if I go blind."

"I think that because this disease usually hits older people, and specifically more women, most of the time it would be like having grandma move in with you when she couldn't see well anymore. I've known people who did this and it sort of worked" I added. Hema listened intently but did not say anything for a while.

"You must have a lot of fear, a lot of fear inside?" she asked, sounding concerned. Obviously it struck both of us simultaneously that neither of us had family here to rely on to take care of us. We had each other though.

"Yes but let's not talk about that now." I wanted to rest in a positive environment and just hoped to get up in the morning without the soreness, and write up the notes of this day's experiences.

We enjoyed the food, then I made some lemon-ginger tea, insisting on needing to move around and do something constructive. I lay down on her on the couch and sort of watched television but mostly listened without looking as my eye was so sore it was hard to keep it open. Just after 10pm my eyes wanted to go to bed and, again, they dragged the rest of me with them uncompromisingly towards complete rest. As we lay there for a while still awake, Hema said,

"There's a reason we came into each other's lives."

"To take care of each other", I replied, and we lay there quietly for a while.

Again she said I must have a lot of fear inside of me, and a lot of emotions. Again I said I did not want to focus on that right now. I wanted peaceful rest, not frightening reflection. We both slept badly, but it was so good to have her there with me.

Sharing Ancient Footprints

The next morning was a nice foggy overcast start to the day. I was pain free and in a much better mood. The fig trees had lush light green leaf buds on them, and the grass in my yard was overgrown from the recent rains and warm weather. Hema called from the road as she was heading towards campus to teach. I thanked her for taking care of me, for which she chastised me. Why was I thanking her so much, she wanted to know? Why could I not thank her if I wanted to? I laughed with her that I would include this moment in my written notes!

I went for a much needed walk in the park by myself. Everywhere around life was about to burst forth into springtime, and the energy of it was contagious. It helped, but I had awoken with the following line clearly on my mind which I repeated and tried to understand as I walked through Battleground Park: "Amidst the footprints of the ancients, there I will lay me down the dreams and sorrows of my heart."

I did not fully understand the line though it inspired me as I walked. I said it over and over in my mind. It made me feel like I was part of something bigger, something with a richer, even ancient, history. Later it made me sad as I read it on the computer screen. Perhaps my mind was thinking back to the people who had gone before me with this disease—the ancients with whom I am now irreversibly connected. After all I had discussed a little of this history of treatment with the nurse and it had struck me how unfortunate people had been before 2005. Perhaps it's a metaphor for inevitability and mortality—I have a sense that I will live a similar life of struggle that others before me had. Perhaps it is a line from a poem I learned as a child, or a line from a song I had not yet written. More likely it had to do with the fact that I was starting to crave connection with others with similar experiences. How did their dreams and sorrows and mortality play out with this disease, and how was it similar to mine? What same quiet, fearful footsteps were we walking? I knew I needed to let these poetics guide me in this desire for connection.

There's Plenty to Be Thankful for

Shortly after the fourth injection, Hema and I began to make concrete plans for a summer trip to both England and India. We would spend time with each other's families, see where we both grew up, and reconnect for a few weeks with our roots, as well as share them with each other. I looked forward to fixing my eyes on my loved ones. I looked forward to gazing at the important places of our childhoods: place of birth, churches/temples, schools, streets and buildings, and sharing these with Hema. I looked forward, as I know she did, to seeing her family, friends, and homeland. We made tentative plans to try to make it to see the Taj Mahal, as well as other memorable places. This would be in many ways, for me at least, primarily a journey in which to relish things through the visual—a time to embrace and share our lives with each other through what, and who, we would see together. Hovering over these plans was the ever present question of how my sight would be the next time we visited these people and places. At this point, I resolved that this nagging reality would only make the experience of this journey sweeter for us.

Just after Easter, we began the process of applying for the visas necessary to make this trip together. Hema was very busy, so I began working on the forms for the visa for me to enter India. I found the Indian visa webpage which included a clear video introduction to the forms and how to complete them. Somehow I missed all of this and ended up battling through the form with no real sense of what I was doing, and cursing that it was unclear and difficult. The first time I completed the online form I had somehow checked yes to indicate that my grandparents were from Pakistan—something that my parents would find amusing. The second time I missed off my middle name. The third time I missed my job title. I had presented myself as working for UNCG but with no specific designation. I also managed to find, and complete, a visa payment form that was entirely different from, and far more expensive than, the one Hema sent me. All in all it was a fiasco, and a waste of a day. Each time the form started from a blank page, saving nothing I had inputted, and I grew angrier by the draft. I was furious at myself when Hema had to sit down at the end of a long day and try to figure out what I should have been doing. I was making more work for her. Eventually, and it did take some time that evening, we laughed and agreed that I would not get frustrated with forms, and would not run with what I thought was correct paper work. I would check with Hema first. She would be in charge of documents and related tasks. Half joking, if she would handle paper work, I offered to cook, clean, and pay for the trip. Also half joking, she asked me to keep going with the list of concessions! I had failed to handle what should be a simple paper work task, but we had succeeded in negotiating task assignments relating to some of the things we would face as we travelled this summer, and throughout life.

The rest of that treatment month felt transitional in a positive way. Change was in the air. It was fully Spring-time and about time to plant vegetables and to get the garden/yard in shape for summer. I was trying to get myself in shape. Throughout the injection period, I had gained weight. Perhaps this was a side effect of the medication, or of my low and fearful spirits. I did not know, but I wanted it to change. I was also doing the tasks necessary to go back as a faculty member in August—choosing text books, and so on. I was transitioning to use the new I-Pad instead of paper text books in my upcoming classes. We were coming out of early spring, and planning the vacations that would punctuate the summer before we were both busy again in the fall. I was also transitioning from a set treatment plan of four injections, to one that would more than likely be ongoing and continuous each month, and that might involve both eyes. During this burst of spring, and because things were so uncertain with the future of my treatment, I had put this out of my mind and did not say much to people about my condition, or how things had declined. Mostly I could not really notice decline, although my left eye sort of nagged me with worry just under the surface of my consciousness, but it was not at the forefront of my everyday thoughts. There were poignant moments though.

Hema had been readying me for the trip to India as I was readying her for the trip to England. We watched some movies that were set in India, as an opportunity for her to clarify and illustrate how things would be. We were describing places and people so that we would understand the cultures, and so that we each felt comfortable with the experiences ahead. While walking at the lake near her apartment one evening, Hema pointed to the people further up the path coming towards us: "See the man with the gray hair ahead? My father's hair is just like that, *fully* white"! She emphasized the word "fully" with a dramatic Indian lilt.

"Oh really?!" I replied, "I can see two people ahead, but not their hair … You can see their hair from here?" I added, surprised at how much detail she could see more than I could.

Hema did not reply, probably shocked by the vivid difference in our ability to see. She could see that there were actually three people, and what their hair looked like, and probably much more about them than I could at that distance.

One early morning in the gym I bumped into a colleague from the anthropology department. She had heard about my eye condition and came over to inquire about how I was doing. She asked if the eyes were stabilized by the treatments, the answer to which I did not really know. She was wishing me well—telling me to be in touch if there was anything I needed, a ride to the store, airport, that sort of thing. It was very nice of her. She then told me that there were a group of people at the conference she had just been to who were interested in research relating to disabilities. I told her that I would definitely be pursuing the topic myself. In fact, I had told Hema that I would dedicate much of the rest of my career to the communicative issues surrounding blindness and vision loss. Susan also thought that would be something I could make a real contribution to. I told her I thought so too, but that it was not really the story I wanted to be telling, but here I was—recognizing that sometimes our stories choose us. Perhaps they do, or perhaps we narrate things that way so that the oddities and capriciousness of fate and life appear to have a grander purpose. The eternal crossroads of choice in how we narrate our experiences is never far away—one way meaning and purpose, another absurdity and despair. Also never far away is the intersection where these two choices often mingle and combine uncomfortably, chaotically, and emotionally.

I bought new sunglasses—a pair of Smith Optics "Guides Choice." They offered full coverage for my eyes, meaning that the sun could not glare over or around the rims when I pushed them up against my face. They also had polarchromic lenses, in amber, which was the perfect color tone for me to see well. The gray clip on's I used for driving and other activities simply flattened the contrasts too much; gray lenses, gray road, many gray cars, meant it was difficult to see and distinguish things well. This was not good, especially while driving. Amber seemed to invigorate images, and the high quality polarization reduced my fear of being out in the bright spring sun. I planned outside activities much less around the dimmer parts of the day, and more around when I wanted to do things. I was thrilled.

On Easter Sunday, midway between the last injection and the next, my dear pal Bud Goodall popped up on Facebook chat—something he rarely did.

"Happy Easter my friend, how are you doing?" He began.

"Happy Easter, doing well. You?" I replied.

"Good enough thanks. Getting new test results this week, so we'll see. How are you 'seeing' things?" He continued.

"Best wishes with the tests. Hoping for good news old luv. Am doing ok … in the eternal 'we'll see what happens by next month' discourse!" I added.

"Thanks! I'm afraid we're in the same 'next month discourse'! But every day is a gift and there's plenty to be thankful for ..." he said.

We went on to talk about summer plans; ours to England and India, theirs to London, Dublin and Edinburgh with side trips as part of a summer abroad program. Indeed we had things to look forward to. I was amazed at how full he had kept his upcoming time. His days were numbered, and he knew it.

"At the end of July I am supposed to be doing a writing workshop in Chapel Hill. Will you be back in Greensboro then?" He asked.

"Yes ... would love to see you, here or in Chapel Hill." I replied.

"Let's plan on it. Assuming our 'discourses' remain stable ..." He joked.

"Haha, yes let's. That would be great. Hope the tests come through good. Discourses are never stable as you know but we'll do it anyway!!" I affirmed.

"Indeed we will. Already looking forward to it ... great chatting with you my friend. I think of you often and always send positive vibes, prayers and best wishes ..." He said.

"You too. Enjoy the day and the Easter chocolate!!" I concluded.

Here we were, playfully connecting our current experiences in order to reconnect our lives and our friendship once again—while helping to create a future tense to our lives, insisting on it actually. We were co-creating and affirming our lives as meaningful and purposeful rather than as spectacles of absurdity and macabre despair. One of the lessons in this difficult experience keeps repeating to teach me that happiness and hopefulness are indeed a narrative enterprise—they are created and maintained through hopeful talk and its close correlates of thought and behavior.

Immediately prior to the fifth injection coming up on April 20th our beloved roses were in full bloom in the garden. They were a joy to both of us, and I could not imagine not being able to see them, or distinguish their exquisite colors. We had deep reds, buttery yellows, bright pinks, and creamy whites. I told a friend that alcohol no longer appealed to me because I wanted to hold onto reality, not escape from it. A rose must be experienced as a rose. I do not think he quite got my meaning, but I know that I did.

· 7 ·

FIFTH INJECTION

April 20th 2012

I sat in the waiting room and realized that, apart from relatives waiting with and for others, I was the youngest person here. Despite this fact I felt quite good about our progress, if a little nervous, waiting for my name to be called. I could just see that the date on my watch was two days off. It probably had been since the end of February. It did not make much difference either way but I corrected it. I checked my cell phone for messages even though I had just done so before I arrived, and generally tried to fill the waiting time with things that told myself I could still see quite well. I think, subconsciously, I did not want to look like the worst case in the room. Perhaps I was saying to myself that I am both here, and not here.

Deeper Characters with Real Lives

The nurse who took me seemed a little annoyed that I did not have much to report for her to write down. It is very difficult to articulate tiny or unnoticeable differences, and there is no training on how to describe clearly as a patient. I kept saying that I thought things were about where they were last time. My eyes felt quite stable. We went through the usual eye tests and dilations, and it turned out that I had bounced back a little to somewhere just under 20/40 and just above 20/50. That was encouraging. I felt that the next line down was only just out of reach. To read the line indicating 20/40 would have been sweet. Anyway, we were quickly on to the picture taking room. Only one picture of each eye was taken, which was fine with me, and I was out into the waiting area in line to see Dr. Sanders. I went to the restroom and on my return there was a couple, Lisa and Vic, sitting next to where I left my phone and sunglasses. We had the same phones and this sparked up a good, if brief, conversation.

"Did you leave your phone"? asked Lisa.

"No I left it here to run to the restroom," I replied.

"You both have the same phones. Why do men like Droid's?" she asked.

"I don't know. I got it because it has the biggest screen when I was looking" I replied.

"Are you from South Africa or London?" Vic asked.

"England" I replied, wondering why those particular choices?

"I work with a guy from South Africa. It's a very similar sounding accent" said Vic.

"Yes it is." I assured.

"What is it that you have with your eyes?" I followed up. I had never asked anyone in this place the question before and had no idea how they would respond.

"He has tears in his retinas. 20/20 vision otherwise but they tear for some reason" explained Lisa. Wow, I thought! What a deep and tragic irony to live with. They also live with as much uncertainty and bad mystery as I do, I thought to myself.

"And then there's the cataracts from all of the laser surgeries he's had" she went on.

I explained what I had.

"Do you have high blood pressure, or what causes that?" Lisa inquired.

"They said it was genetic. No one has it in my family but …"

"Well it could have skipped for generations, you never know" Vic intervened.

"I know yes … scary isn't it?" I added hinting at the emotional toll of eye diseases that we no doubt share.

"Yes it is. Makes you realize how important your eyes are. Everyone's are. Everyone uses their eyes for what they do" Vic said.

"If my retinas detach completely I'm done. *Blind*" he added, clarifying the emotional burden he was also feeling towards the uncertainty and risk he also faced every day.

"I hope the best for you with them" I said.

"And you too" he responded warmly.

We all introduced ourselves by name, and talked briefly about what we did for a living.

"I've done hunting and fishing all my life and I'm a motor cycle enthusiast. I can't imagine not being able to do those things." Vic picked up the conversation. I could tell there was as much worry behind his comment, as I had for the potential loss of the passions and hobbies that were part of my identity.

"I understand. I do. Every day is a blessing isn't it?" I responded surprising myself with this statement.

"Yes it is" they both immediately replied.

"Hey," I said, as if drawing them into a private moment and to lighten the mood, "do these people talk to the DMV"?!

We all laughed.

Lisa went on to tell me how her eyes were also right on the legal border, but when she went to get her license renewed recently the eye testing machine was not working properly, so the DMV person waived that part. She passed the test for another ten years. We laughed again. She had made it over an important border in her life, undetected! Then my name was called by Loren and I was off to wait for Dr. Sanders. I could tell we all enjoyed the conversation. It was the first time I had talked to someone who has lived through something similar. He had similar fears and hopes if a different disease and, again, it made me want to hear more about the existential experience of vision loss that others also lived through and with.

Dr. Sanders was very upbeat about how much of an impact the treatments had by this point. He was right to continue with the injections into the right eye—it was almost inactive except for a couple of microscopic spots. He was also right to not begin a course of treatment in the left eye—there was no activity to be seen in it. Good job all round! We all felt good about things. He said that we would move the injections now to once every six weeks instead of every four. We were not ceasing the process, but dropping back to less frequent injections was welcome news for all of us. I told him I was beginning a research program to explore my experience of struggling with vision loss and its impact on communication, and that I would like to connect to the experiences of others also. I tried to explain what a "communication approach" meant—that I was interested in its impact on communication, and the role of relationships in shaping the experience of the process of vision loss. I do not think he could quite see the central question I was driving at, and I was not articulating it well, but he was interested in the prospect:

"Well, at some point would it be possible to connect with some of your other patients for interviews?" I asked.

"Yes, we could provide a surrogate whereby we can contact patients and have them contact you if they want to participate" he explained.

"Ok great, well that would be good in terms of protecting their privacy, etc. Yes I will have to go through IRB approval on the research design so it's early days on that at this point" I added, thinking I was rambling a bit.

"If there are only a few patients, it might be an issue in terms of their traceability back to your clinic ..." I was a little disoriented, and was trying to say there might be an issue with the anonymity of the subjects but I couldn't quite get there clearly. He picked up on what I was trying to say.

"We're talking about a large number of people! This procedure for WMD is a big part of our practice." He clarified.

"OK great," I started filling in more of the details, and thinking out loud about the research possibilities. But we needed to get back to the business of the moment ...

"Let's talk about this when the research design matures. I don't want to take your time here." He moved us into the preparation phase for the injections, assisted by the lovely Loren.

My mind was buzzing with the prospects for this research, as he was directing me through the injection procedure.

"Look left" he said. I didn't respond, still looking right, towards where he was positioned.

"Look left, look over at Loren"

"AHH," I said, "Yes the *other* left!"

I quickly remembered to open my left eye and look at Loren's upturned index finger with both eyes. Otherwise I would have been focused with my whole vision through my right eye at the needle coming at my eye—which was definitely not a good idea!

"You're safe, you're safe," he said calmly, as the relatively painless needles were going in and out of my eye.

After the injection I told Loren how important her holding her index finger up was to making the experience less frightening. She was glad. I told her that Matt wiggled his finger when he assisted. She said she would do that too if requested but that sometimes people moved their eyes to the wiggle, which was not good. They told me that Amanda, who had taken care of me several times, had her baby and that everything was fine. This was a happy visit all round. Good news seems to attract good news. Dr. Sanders planned to see me in six weeks and was gone to help another patient. Loren washed and disinfected my eye, and told me she would love to travel to my native England. We also talked a little about her merged family of six brothers and sisters. She told me she did not want children, which I had a hard time believing. She asked me if I liked to write a lot—a response to our discussion of research earlier. This slight deepening of all of our relationships beyond the sterile medical procedure into more personal sharing, albeit in a compressed time frame, felt reassuring. We were becoming more real as characters for each other in this common treatment story—with dimensions of background lives, dreams, hopes, likes and dislikes, and so on, being added with each visit.

The Care of Help

I took my usual route home, glad at first that it was overcast. I soon realized that this white cloud cover that diffused the bright sunlight was actually more difficult to drive in. The brightness was all around instead of localized mostly near where the sun was coming from. I made it home, thankful for the safety. I ate and then slept for a couple of hours. Hema called and I relayed the good news about the treatment period being moved to six weeks rather than four, and the relative stability during this month. My eyes were less tired than normal as they only took two photographs. We still planned to stay home that evening, to allow me to recover in peace and quiet.

I wanted a glass of wine, and some chocolate, to celebrate after the lovely meal Hema prepared. We might also rent a movie there. She also needed to pick up something so we started to drive to the grocery store. As we were driving, she announced that she wanted to go by Kohl's to pick up something for a friend's one year birthday party the next afternoon. I said no—wanting to stay away from people and their germs. She was disappointed, but swung the car towards the grocery store. I relented, feeling selfish, and told her it would be fine to go to Kohl's, and that it would not take long to pick up an outfit for the toddler. She was hesitant, but I pushed her to change directions towards Kohl's. There was a grocery store next door where we could get the other items—a reasonable compromise. When we got to Kohl's it was quiet, and I felt fine. However, when I found out we were actually shopping for three different children, one for tomorrow and two for nieces we would see on our trip in July, I was annoyed again. Why were we doing this now? I tried to be accommodating, and not get angry, which only made her anxious, and I know she enjoyed having me there as she picked out things for the children of our families. As she searched for the clothes, I drifted off on my own to not be in the way. The outfits she settled on were cute. She would apparently save more if she bundled the purchases together. I went with it, not really understanding how that worked, and we were soon in the grocery store. I had wanted a really nice glass of wine to celebrate the good news, but had to settle for the better option they had in the fridge, which was not very good. We rented "The Help" and were soon on our way home. I was glad we had both picked up what we wanted and chosen what turned out to be a good movie together. I had been pushed out of my post-injection routine and it worked out fine, and I did not catch any terrible virus at either stores.

For the rest of that evening we relaxed and watched the film. It struck me how the movie brought to life the fact that not only did these black women have to serve white people, but as they did so, they were constantly performing the idea that serving them properly was their life purpose. They had to look like they meant it; that they *wanted* to serve, and that pleasing the other was crucial to their own happiness. They had to look like they loved the people they served. Perhaps this is a historical root of what we now know as performing "good service"—something for which America is well known. I do not know if there is any connection, but the story of these poor people and their everyday joys, struggles, and resistance tactics took me away from my troubles, and kept us both enthralled. When it ended, I was ready to go to bed with the hope that tomorrow the soreness would lessen.

On our walk, a day or so later, Hema revealed that she wanted to play tennis and learn golf together. I was happy that she was optimistic and wanted to do these things with me. I was not sure if I could, or how well I could, but I was willing to try at some point if things stayed stable with my eyes. I was a little nervous that we might be slipping from assuming a narrative of "decline" to an unrealistic one of "overcoming and back to normality", but I left the topic alone.

In early May, BBC America ran a very short clip as human interest teaser right before commercial break on the success of an experiment to implant digital eyes into two patients. Granted, the brief story was designed to keep people tuned in until "the other side" of the break as they currently said, but it was good to see something vision related on the news. Although the patients were only able to see light from dark at this point in the experimentation process, it made me glad that surely people out there were working on vision problems, and stood to reap the rewards necessary to stimulate the research in the US. With ageing populations in many industrialized nations, technology as well as medication designed for vision loss and blind people, would surely be a growth industry. Someone out there was seeing the opportunity and the need and, although the profit motive was obvious, it was a good feeling to see things happening for blind people.

DC and Early Summer

In mid-May we went to DC for a long weekend getaway for Hema to relax after her final grades were turned in for the year. For me it would be an interesting trip in terms of revisiting the gem and mineral collection—something I had on my list of things to see. It would also give me an opportunity to revisit a place, this time walking around experiencing the place from a low-vision perspective.

We travelled by metro while in DC. Between the dimly lit small station-signs visible only when right in a station, the inaudible audio directions and announcements, difficult ticketing procedures that required human assistance even for fully sighted people, and the metro line information that is dependent wholly on color perception and differentiation (red, blue, green), I would give the metro a C- for low-vision design accommodation. It would have been easy to add redundancy to the line information with shapes—red is the triangle line for example, but this was not thought of in the planning stage. Clear and large signage was also apparently not a priority. It took a couple of trips but Hema soon got that hang of the metro for us. If I were alone it would have been very difficult.

It was a hot humid and relentlessly bright day when we walked for hours around the mall. Hema was excited to see the monuments and landmarks. We settled on the natural science museum for a tour—mostly at my prompting. We made our way to the Harry Winston gallery which housed some beautiful gems and jewelry and, in particular, showcased the Hope Diamond. We waited our turn to look at the unique gem through the Perspex case, which was grimy with hand prints and human breath. Neither of us were particularly moved or awed by the diamond and its opulent setting. It did not communicate hope in any way to us if that was the intent behind the name. The historical information was too small to read. Hema actually thought it looked black, which would have decreased its value. I have to say I thought the diamond as well as the diamond encrusted setting was beautiful, but just that—a beautiful piece of jewelry.

We joined the flow of the large crowd circling around the other gems displayed in the room. Hema found a sapphire piece whose stones matched her engagement ring—albeit much larger. She was thrilled by this. This fleeting connection to the named gem in the case was probably the highlight for both of us. There was not much time to pause or reflect among the crowd, so we did a quick tour of the whole room without talking much at all. We enjoyed the gems and mineral specimens, everything was of the highest quality and rarity, but it was not the amazing experience I had years before. I was not gushing over the faceted kyanite, or mesmerized by the perfect tourmaline crystals as I had several years before. I was not trying to stay in the room as long as possible, despite the pleas of friends for us to move on. I was more excited about having my picture taken in front of the huge elephant in the atrium, and wondering if I would get this close to a live one on the upcoming trip to India this summer. Walking among the largely African tigers, lions, hippos, and the cute bush pig with it curiously elegant feet, I wondered on what my eyes would delight in India. Although I could see the gem and jewelry objects well, my interests and passions were shifting with my eyes as I looked to the future and somewhat away from the things that defined my interests in the past. It was good to get some clarity on this, as I had wondered with some anticipation at how I would react to the world class gem collection. It was impressive and beautiful. It spoke to me again, but in some odd way it had ceased to speak *of* me.

On the second day, we were tired from the relentless walking of the first day and the lack of rest from the strep throat we were both recovering from. Hema's coughing was so bad I had grabbed a couple of hours of sleep on the bathroom floor on top of a couple of spare blankets—something I had not done since I shared a conference hotel room with my dear pal Bud Goodall who was an Olympian snorer! So, starting out tired, we took the tourist open top bus tour. It was another hot sunny muggy day and the top deck was comfortable only when the bus was moving. I could not imagine how people did this in August in DC when this was only May. We enjoyed seeing the sights and hearing the brief history of them. I was glad to see her enchanted by the buildings, and distracted from work for a while. We got off the bus at the white house and sat on benches across from the perimeter fence. I wanted to stretch out under a tree and sleep but Hema insisted on sitting on a bench and looking across at the White House. Hema imagined President Obama making a surprise appearance, and we took pictures with the White House in the background. Pure tourist fun! We walked back down Pennsylvania Avenue to Judiciary Square where thousands of police officers from around the US were gathering for a parade—all wearing their home jurisdiction uniforms. Hema, in particular, enjoyed walking around in a city for a change. Everywhere we travelled she wanted to move there! Could I get a job here and we could live somewhere nice like Rosslyn where we were staying, she wondered. I could not imagine getting around and living in a place like DC. The traffic is awful and the metro mediocre at best for someone with low vision. I did not say this, of course, but kept the thought to myself. She loved to imagine, and I enjoyed hearing her dream out loud.

By the end of the day, even though I wore a sun hat and good sunglasses, when I closed my eyes back in the room, my retinas were glowing a dull red like warm coals. They were exhausted and hurting from the full day of bright sunlight. I needed a hot shower, a cold beer, and a warm bed. In an effort to make sure we slept better, Hema had thoughtfully negotiated our move to a hypoallergenic room just down the hall. It really made a difference for us in that she coughed much less that night. The new room, a hot shower, some food, two pints of cold Stella, and a shot of Benadryl, and I was oblivious to noises—coughing, snoring or otherwise. We slept well and my eyes felt rested the next morning.

We were having a good time but I was spending money on this trip at an alarming rate, and we had a big trip coming up. I was nervous about making it into the fall with some savings left, paying off the expensive upcoming travel, and building things back up financially after a year at half pay while on research leave. All of this was set against the backdrop of fear over my eye conditions. Everywhere along the path of everyday life seemed to be the perennial tug between "do it while you can" and "be cautious for the future". Balancing these voices is perhaps one of the keys to happy living, and it was an even more poignant balancing act with a progressive eye disease.

Upon my return to town I had my Indian visa waiting, which we were thrilled about. It had come through in a matter of a few days while we were gone to DC. We were just waiting now for Hema's UK visa to come so that we were covered for that part of the trip as well. I also had an email from my rock cutting pal Tim in Georgia, firming up the invite for us to go there sometime in June. His email contained the following touching statement as a response to my news to him that things seemed relatively stable with regards to the decline of my eyes: "… Glad to hear it about the eyes, we had the whole congregation praying for you (I have not turned into zealot, but we are trying to make a communion service once a month, and for important stuff I do put in prayer requests) …"

My friend had the whole church praying for me and I had never met any of them. How wonderful people can be when they organize for good and kind things. I was grateful and moved by the gesture. I sent thanks to them all through Tim. Perhaps their good works were helping as I was feeling quite positive about things as the next injection drew closer (May 25th).

Our friend Suresh, who took us out to for a wonderful Thai meal at Thai Square in Rosslyn had asked Hema why we flew to DC when it was only a five hour drive. He did not know about my eyes. She explained that my eye condition made it difficult for me to drive in unfamiliar places, and he immediately asked her to have me send information on my condition to him via email, which I did. It turned out his wife was an ophthalmologist with a research as well as clinical background, and would be happy to connect with me on the topic—perhaps providing some insights I did not have, or a lead to more understanding. I would truly appreciate any useful information. I sent my information and awaited their reply. His ophthalmologist wife was in India for a wedding so it would take some time to hear back. I actually never heard back on the eye information he said he might be able to get for me. Rather, instead, we heard that he and his wife were likely splitting and he was retiring back to India. She had other concerns more pressing than helping his friends.

My "Welcome Back" and Workplace Worry

Right before the next injection, I picked up my key to my new office in the renovated Curry building on campus. I was excited to see the renovation job. Curry offices had more character than Ferguson, and more traffic/energy. The department in Ferguson had no classrooms so there was very little student traffic, apart from people coming by with a problem or to drop off papers. I had asked for the office close to the end of my time as head so that it would be waiting for me when I returned. It would be a fresh location to come back to. As I walked in I was stunned to see the most beat up, scratched, mismatched and incomplete old furniture that I had ever seen in an office on campus. I could not believe it. I was speechless, hurt, and then angry. I walked back to the Ferguson building to catch the new department head. I explained to him that I had been left junk for furniture and asked if he could purchase at least a new desk. He looked at me and simply asked, "So is the furniture scratched, what exactly is wrong with it?" I was speechless again. He looked at me as if to say, what are you complaining about? He wandered back to his office with a nice big mug of coffee in his hand, and that was that.

After eight years foraging for resources for faculty, including him, to meet their needs I am treated this way? I walked away thinking … "So, I would be the only tenure line faculty member with junk for furniture?" I just could not believe it. I thought about it on the way home and hoped against all hope that the technology I had just received to help me navigate my sight limitations—a large computer screen, and an I-Pad for my text books, was not being held against me. I hoped this was not a "hey you just got some new things so get to the back of the line" moment. Surely those items would be viewed as separate to the request for newer furniture. I wanted to address these issues with my department head—the inequality of the furniture, and the potentially difficult issue of having accommodations count as purchases that pushed me to the back of the line for other things that everyone else had. I was so stunned that I said nothing. Perhaps there simply was no money, as he said, but there would be come July and there was no indication that I would get furniture equivalent to my colleagues even then. At least something from this century would have been acceptable.

Perhaps I should have spoken up. Perhaps I would have been perceived as a former head trying to bully new furniture out of the new guy. Perhaps I was being "put in my place." Perhaps the staff would have resented me getting furniture when they had not had a raise in several years. Perhaps there were just other priorities for what little money there was—other needs, louder or more favored voices. I had no idea what web of interpretations formed the backdrop to this scenario. I just left it alone. I was disappointed and hurt, seeing this as my "welcome back" but I said nothing and resolved to buy some new furniture for myself, and just get on with things.

Later that evening I was joking with a friend on the phone that if my eyes declined rapidly I would not know I had lousy office furniture as I would not be able to see it, and so it was not really a problem! The humor helped, and the moment of anger passed, but it did raise questions for me about how "accommodations" would be perceived in my workplace. What was the real level of sensitivity and support for disability, and how would purchases relating to my vision problems actually be perceived by those with power over me? This was a question I had never even thought of before, and now it was suddenly central to my return to campus.

The day before my next injection I scrubbed the house clean and cooked several dishes so that I would come home to a clean house after the injections, and we would not have to cook for a couple of days at least. It was mid-May, and exactly a year since this story began in earnest when I got a reminder postcard to come and have my regular eye test. I reminded myself that one of the recommendations of the online advice is to keep up with regular eye exams. Part of me felt that I had regular exams—much more detailed and comprehensive than the optometrist—every time I went for injections, but I also knew that I needed to make an appointment anyway. Perhaps my prescription had also changed, and they would focus on that important issue for me. I resisted and delayed for three weeks, not wanting more frustrating letter recognition tests, dilation, or more lights and flashes of photographs into my eyes. Perhaps, I thought, with all of the letter tests I had been through and those to come, I could begin to memorize them for when I redid my driver's license test in a few years.

YEAR 2

Mid-May 2012 to Mid-May 2013

· 8 ·

SIXTH INJECTION

May 25th 2012

"I'm thrilled. This is the best possible scenario! Your right eye has responded to treatment very well. It's the best structurally now that it will ever be. The edema is gone, and there's no fluid or bleeding in either eye." Dr. Sanders said enthusiastically, and a great start to the year it was.

"You did great!" He added.

"Wow, that's great! Thanks for all of your help" I responded, lifted by the positive evaluation. His decisions throughout the process—pushing me to begin treatment immediately back in December when we could easily have put it off until the new year; deciding how often I needed injections; holding off on injections in the left-eye when he could easily have prescribed that at one time when it looked like it was starting to have problems, all played an important part in the current level of success we shared in this moment. We were sitting in one of the now familiar consulting rooms looking at the digital images of my retinas on the monitor screen on the wall that Dr. Sanders was clicking through, back and forth. The materials for this month's injections were laid out neatly on the counter to my right.

"Well, whatever you're doing … I don't know … praying … whatever it is, keep it up!"

"I will Doc., thanks." He must be a religious man, I thought to myself. I thought so, for some reason, all along.

"We will always have to keep an eye on things, but let's have you back in eight weeks instead of six for the next treatment. You'll miss us, I know, but you'll have to find something else to do!" he joked.

The good news was sweet, but almost as surreal as the moment I got the bad news a year or so ago, because it was both surprising and hard to grasp exactly what it meant at that time, or what it would mean in the longer term. Enjoy the moment, I thought to myself, and I pushed the worry aside for another day and time.

These words shared with Dr. Sanders marked a very positive start to year two of this experience. Although—worryingly—the treatment went on after the normal course of four injections, the two extra ones I had had so far seemed to have made the difference in stabilizing things. Something in my eyes was stubbornly trying to express itself at the expense of my sight—a side effect or some reaction in a causal chain that we did not quite understand. Actually, we did not talk about causality much at all, which I would have liked to do, but I do not think he had a clear sense of why this was happening to me. Everything focused on what the medication was doing to stop the immediate decline. Nevertheless, it looked like whatever it was had finally relenting to the "wonder drug" (Avastin) as Dr. Sanders called it last December when he began injections. Would year two be a better one? I hoped it would be, and that I could get back as close as possible to the "normal" that for a year now had been steadily, and frighteningly, slipping away.

"Now let's get you ready for the injection this time …"

I was ready. First came the numbing drops, then the eye-lid clip which held my eye open and prevented me from blinking. Then came the slightly painful pinch of the numbing injection. It was always good when this part was over. Loren and Dr. Sanders switched the lights down low and were gone to another room, to help someone else, while my eye was numbing in readiness for the Avastin shot. As I waited alone in the darkened room for the numbing injection to do its job, I enjoyed looking at the slowly rotating images from nature that were showing on the monitor screens in the room. Seeds, snowflake crystals, cells of various kinds, and other microscopic images of the wonders of nature and life in clear, high definition, were truly beautiful and relaxing to watch. My mind drifted back to the waiting area where I sat just a few minutes ago and witnessed another pleasurable microcosm of life—a beautiful conversation …

It was rare for people to chat as they waited but an elderly, and very well dressed, African-American couple came into the waiting area and insisted on disrupting the pensive silence. I noticed their dress was coordinated, with black and purple as central themes. Were they going somewhere afterwards, or did they dress formally for the Doctor visit? I had no idea, and could not think of an easy or polite way to ask. As they sat down, the man said to the rest of us jokingly, "So, can you see?!"

The three of us waiting for treatment all laughed, immediately aware of what connected us in this place, and of how difficult a question this was to answer—there was no simple yes/no answer to this question for any of us anymore, and I suspect he knew this. It was an inside joke doubling as a conversational opener. The couple proceeded to chat with the white couple who were approximately the same age sitting next to them; finding commonalities, affirming their choice of Dr. Sanders as an excellent retina specialist, their common distrust of the profit motive of much of the medical and pharmaceutical world, and so on. Interspersed with this, the African-American couple teased each other playfully in the same way that Hema and I often did. The wife told a story of how her husband put off, and put off, seeking treatment until he had lost most of the sight in one of his eyes. If she had not pushed him who knows if he would have come at all, or be able to see at all by now? She pointed out that he was still able to read the newspaper better than she could, which confounded her. (What people sometimes do not realize is that vision loss can be such a specific thing. It is often quite nuanced. He may be able to read the paper well, but not recognize people in a photograph or see road signs to drive a car safely, for example.) I smiled to myself. I was thankful for Hema, as I am sure he was for her, for pushing me to get help, and for teasing me as she often did. "What am I going to do with this guy?" I could almost hear her saying as she shook her head. And, like the African-American lady sitting across from me, this was most likely simply another way of indirectly saying, "Where would you be without me?" or "If only you would listen to me all of the time …" Both women had a fair point, and I suspected we both knew it! Was putting off going to the Doctor more of a male thing to do as her talk hinted? I remember that my mother was just as bad in her day—not wanting to "bother the Doctor." I do not know, but I know Hema pushed me frequently to get help and resolve things, and I was quietly grateful as I sat there waiting for the Avastin injection.

Dr. Sanders returned and with the bright lights back on, and the next injection smoothly lining up, I was very much back in the present moment: "So are you ready for the easy part …?" He asked.

I was ready for the injection and now, numbed and relaxed, he was right—it really was the easy part. The actual Avastin injection was almost painless, and over in just a few seconds. There was always a moment of inner panic as the needle came towards the eye from the right, but Lauren's finger off to the left once again helped divert my gaze away from the needle—from horror to beauty is always a good trade. I knew she must have seen some interesting emotions in patient's faces in that existential moment of injection—fear, dread, sorrow, perhaps even anger—I never asked her, but looking back I wished I had.

The muted buzz around the doctor's office was of Memorial-Day weekend plans of which we had none of interest to anyone else. Lorren said she did not have big plans either and that she would just hang out in town. Hema was recovering from ingrown toenail surgery, and I liked to minimize plans right after an injection in case my eye was sore, and to avoid infections. We planned to just enjoy being together to take care of each other. Besides, neither of us grew up with the memorial-day rituals of going to the coast as people did here. I was happy for the quiet, stress-free roads around town for the long weekend. As my eyes got worse it seemed that Greensboro's drivers also got worse, but I knew it was not them, it was me experiencing fear.

I made my next appointment with Clare at the front desk. She gave me the closest available day and early morning time to eight weeks from now (July 27th). In my mind I calculated that we would be safely home from our trip to England and India before the next injections. Perfect timing! She reminded me physically of a college girlfriend, oddly also named Clare, who I had dated and then lived with briefly at the end of my college days. Perhaps she reminded many of us middle-aged and older male patients of a college girlfriend from long ago! When I checked in an hour or so ago I joked with her about her Reese's stash just visible in her part opened drawer. She told me, quietly, that she snacks all day as it helps pass the time. I think the staff now recognized me, and were a little friendlier each time I went. I knew that behind the professional comportment they had dull days that dragged as we all did. I imagined she was glad it was Friday and the start of a long early summer weekend. We exchanged good weekend wishes and I was on my way to my car. I called Hema and told her I was done with my treatment and was on my way out, so that she knew I was ok, and so she could warm up our lunches.

I walked out into blazing May sunshine. It was the start of Memorial-Day weekend and, as I headed directly to my car, the sun was high in the sky, hot on the ground, and bright in the eyes. The drive home was painful. Every light seemed to turn red on me, and I struggled to look up at the lights against the raw bright daylight just behind them. Cursing loudly and angrily each time a light turned red and delayed me, I was glad Hema was not in the car to witness this. She really did not like angry cursing as it reminded her of her ex-husband, and her father before that, and therefore made her feel unsafe and afraid. I think my anger was based on fear and vulnerability, just as her reaction was, because I just wanted to get home to safety, and it did not seem like the traffic lights were on my side. How quickly the fear had changed me from just a few moments ago, I reflected. I was shouting wildly at lights that seemed to be consciously victimizing me. Despite this stressful journey home I was relieved, and glad, that things seemed to be leveling out with my eyes. We would not know for how long, but that question needed to be pushed back from my thoughts for now. It was a weekend to enjoy life, good news, and the coming of summer. A plateau—a reprieve from decline—is infinitely preferable to a downturn, and should be enjoyed as a moment, *in the moment*.

Several people have asked me why I do not just ask friends for a ride home, and my answer is always that it would be inconvenient for them. I never know when I will get out of there, and this makes it awkward for people to coordinate leaving work to drop me home. At the same time, on some level, I also enjoyed knowing that I could get home by myself. I was still relatively independent, and that was really important to me. The injection itself did not affect driving, it was just the dilation that meant the world was too bright, but I figured out ways to work around that. I stuck to my well known path home in which there were no left turns out onto roads, at least not without traffic lights.

When I got home, Hema had put together a lovely lunch of prior cooked food which we ate and then I went to bed, and immediately to sleep, for what turned out to be my usual two hours. Kindly, she closed all the doors to make sure I was not disturbed. I was safe in her care. I awoke ready for a good strong cup of tea. The world outside still seemed unnaturally bright, as I was a little dilated still. Do people really have any idea how bright and powerful the sun is I wondered? Just a slight adjustment of the pupil kept us all in balance with its enormous power. It could give life and it could destroy. No wonder many people over the millennia have worshiped the sun, I thought as I sat in the chair with my tea. It seemed godlike in its powers and relentless omnipresent cycle. Some seemed to be chosen to be able to soak up its love, and others were hurt by it even in short bursts. In this moment of tender dilation, the sun just seemed to me to be so massive and supernaturally powerful.

We waited until 6 pm to go to the store and buy some wine and chocolate to celebrate. We actually only had a little of each that evening as we were not used to either one of late. Part of me wondered why these were still celebratory for us. We could replace them with something healthier and not miss these sugary treats. Processed sugar was on my no-no list, and yet its reward association still ran deep for me. We relaxed in the evening and watched the movie, "All the pretty horses." It was an epic tale of love found, and love lost again. I was thankful to be here safe on the couch with my sweetheart instead of wandering around Mexico and Texas surviving the tribulations that Matt Damon's character endured. As usual, he was great in his role. I was struck by how relentlessly bright the sun must be in that dry, scorched, rocky looking part of the world. I wondered how many blue-eyed cowboys (as well as sailors and farmers in other places) who worked their lives out in the blazing sun lived through maculopathy and suffered in silence, many not even having a name for it, and certainly no treatment options.

After the movie, I tried to watch "Fashion Police" featuring Joan Rivers and friends. I always got a kick out of her. I was a bit of a "Joan Ranger" as her fans are called! I made it half-way through the show and my eyes were just "done" for the day. They dragged me to bed while Hema switched to working on her online summer school course until after midnight. She was staying in the spare room because her feet were so vulnerable and tender after just having toe-mail surgery, as was my eye. What a pair we made! I did not hear her go to bed, as I was asleep as soon as my head touched the pillow, but at 2:30 am I was awoken by her gently calling my name. Apparently I had woken up the 24th time that she called for me! I was in a deep sleep, even—allegedly—snoring louder when she was calling my name some of the first 23 times! She had a nightmare, probably from the pain medication, and wanted me to comfort her. She came back to bed with me and I could not get back to sleep, but I did not complain. Although I lost half a night's sleep there was nothing pressing the next morning, and my eye felt ok, so I made a conscious effort not to get upset. In the morning I got up, went for a walk in the park, then to the Fresh Market where I picked up croissants and a bunch of flowers and came home to make a nice brunch for Hema. She was thrilled that I remembered that she wanted brunch on Saturday morning (she had mentioned croissants for a few days now—perhaps hinting) and, as ever, she was thrilled to get flowers from me (she bought them for me just as often). It was a weekend to be enjoyed as we took care of each other. It was not without a few fussy moments, as we were used to our own space and routines, but we were there for each other.

Sharing and Savoring Good News

After brunch I chatted with Bud Goodall on Facebook. I told him I joined him in his recent good news about his cancer with my good news about my eye treatment. He was pleased for me, as I was for him. I told him that if he could not make it to North Carolina in July as planned for a workshop he was giving at Chapel Hill we would come out to see him, Sandra, and Nic, in Arizona. He liked the idea. I joked with him that these days, given my eye trouble, he might be able to beat me at pool. He responded that didn't he always beat me? I replied that he could rewrite history a little if he wanted to, and that he deserved to do that. In other words, no, he did not beat me at pool very often back years ago when we used to play regularly! He told me he did not rewrite history but just edited out the bad and boring parts, and that he got that from Elmore Leonard. We joked on until he needed to go and make breakfast. Standing on the tile floor of his kitchen was hard for him, but he was off to cook as he always loved to do. Savoring the simple moments was a joy we both shared in our time of tribulations. We wished each other good Memorial-Day weekends, and signed off.

Shortly after this conversation, I wrote a brief entry for a Festschrift some people were putting together in his honor. I included his Elmore Leonard inspired approach to editing one's life story in my entry, as something that captured the essence of Bud. He always chose the happy and interesting, over the bad and boring—it was the basis of his positivity and happiness, and an admirable habit of being. The title of my short essay was "Intersecting narratives—positive communication." Simply, there were some people in my life who, when their paths crossed with mine, it always led to positive communication and the good things that came from that. Bud was one of those people for me and, no doubt, for many others. The article completed by June 1st was the first time I had written about my vision loss explicitly for something that would be published. I was happy to do so and thought, perhaps, something good might come of the commitment to voice the experience, and share it with others. The deeper lesson that it is the intersections of one's life story with certain people that creates and releases positives into one's life, was one I would think and write more about in future I thought. It was certainly something I would talk about in my upcoming fall class entitled, "Positive Communication."

The after effects of this injection seemed less pronounced than for previous ones. Perhaps the good news helped to deflect from them. Perhaps it was because it was longer than usual since the last one. The next day the soreness and pain seemed less troubling than usual and my eye was not as bloodshot as it usually was. I was thankful for it all. We enjoyed taking care of each other. Hema was protective of her tender and painful feet. She got nervous whenever I was near them. She actually got very frightened when I reached for one of her feet to hold it. I told her that the fear she had in that moment was the same fear I had when she came close to my eye in the days immediately after my injections. I could see her thinking about the analogy. She loved to grab my face, an Indian expression of affection, but I blocked her from doing this when my eye was tender and vulnerable. She would say that she was not going to hurt my eye but, for me, that was not the point. It was a natural protective reaction. She often took this the wrong way, as if I did not trust her. As she reacted the same way over her feet, I joked with her that we had just had a "teachable moment" which made her want to grab my face all the more, but she could not catch me—I had one-over on the monkey (one of my pet names for her) and she knew it!

I had emailed a few people with the good news from my doctor's visit and several wrote back with congratulations. Art, had been through heart tests recently and came out of it with happy news that he just needed to work on wellness and fitness, and that the test result that worried him had been a false positive. Along with Bud's dramatically lower "count" relating to his cancer, this was good news all round. I think we all felt like we were "beating the odds"—luck, fortune, grace, fate, who knows? It depends how you choose to narrate the story. Steve captured these common happy vibes cheerfully in the following impromptu poem:

> "Pete's peepers and Art's heart are reason enough to
> spit against the wind
> and laugh
> hysterically at foiled fate
> as it crawls back to hell's gate
> a loser"
> (Email May 25, 2012)

Art reminded us that Steve also needed to share his "heart news" when it came through after the next round of tests, and he agreed to keep us posted. Friendship and health were becoming intimately woven together for us as a band of friends. Sharing health news and encouragement were becoming a valuable part of our friendships, as had sharing work and other life news over the years. A couple of weeks later Steve completed more tests and reported, happily, that his heart also was doing fine.

Playfully too, that Saturday afternoon (the day after the injections), Hema teased me that my bachelor life was over. She was already planning how to move the bedrooms and office around for when she might move-in. The bigger room would become an office for both of us, and the current office would become the spare room which would be further from our bedroom than it currently is. If we could not move houses for a while, then she was going to reorganize the space to work better for two people, and for two people who might have parental and family guests at some point in the near future from England or India … she had a plan! And the future oriented positive talk was comforting to me, although I was not sure how productive a shared office would be for us! Still, we were not reorganizing for imminent disability as we could quite easily have been at this point but, rather, for happiness together. Perhaps there would be a mix of both at some point but, for now, we focused on the positives of mapping out some desired elements of a common future story—although I was always aware, just behind the talk, that the map would be different from the territory we imagined.

Somehow it seemed like a significant moment the next weekend when I found myself in Wal-Mart with Hema buying storage bags for clothes—the kind that shrink as you vacuum the air out of them. We bought some "travel size" ones for our upcoming trip together but, with the "jumbo" ones, perhaps we were also planning for the efficiency needed to both live in my small (formerly) bachelor pad!

Just a few days after Memorial-Day weekend Doc Watson, the famous blind musician from North Carolina, died. He was blind from early in his life but went on to become an extraordinarily innovative and influential musician in country and blue-grass music. He had apparently told one interviewer that if he was not blind he would probably have been a car mechanic, and would have been just as happy. What an amazing and inspiring attitude to life and to blindness. He was going to love life, and be happy, whether he was blind or not. I paused that day and wondered what gave him this positivity. Perhaps he felt fortunate despite his blindness, and thankful looking back in his later years at having a full and happy family and artistic life despite the humble beginnings he never forgot. I strongly suspected that he felt blessed to have had close family around him throughout his life—something neither Hema nor I had, but we would be that for each other as much as we could.

By early June my eyes felt more stable than they had in a year. I could not detect much, if any, decline. There were still times when I had to wait for my eyes to clunk (silently) into focus when dealing with smaller details, especially if I got up and moved around and then sat back down to read, or write, or watch television. My eyes would be fuzzy from the momentary activity. Perhaps this was a momentary change related to blood pressure. My hope was that they would continue to clunk back into focus. If the time came when they stopped doing this, I knew things would never be the same again. I think the brighter evenings made a difference to my level of comfort while driving. I was not driving into glaring headlights on dark nights at this time of year. We were nearing the summer solstice and the longest day and, although there was much very bright sunshine at times during the afternoons, the conditions were so much better than the dark of winter. Perhaps too I had gotten used to, and adapted for, where I was in my decline. I did not, for example, feel like panicking if I could not tell how close or far a car in front of me was. I just learned to figure it out and trust that I would be ok if I always put caution first. Every time I drove my old Benz I felt lucky to be driving. The recent plateau enabled me to adjust and be calmer about my eye problems. Perhaps it was also the impending vacations where we would get to meet and spend time with both our families. All in all, I was feeling good about things and positive about life. I think Hema knew this, and I could sense that she relaxed more too. She talked about future plans and dreams more, which I knew made her happy. She loved to dream out loud, and I was glad she did.

Adaptation and Self-Advocacy

I had recently gotten an I-Pad, primarily to help me with reading work related journal and book materials. I had also gotten an I-Pod for Christmas from Hema. The I-Pod had sat in my home office for a little over five months without me using it at all. It just felt like too much of a struggle to get to know it, and my patience was very limited with gadgets. My I-Pad had sat in my office for about a month when I suddenly felt a surge of interest to get to know how to use these devices. I wanted to take the I-Pad on our upcoming trip so I could take notes, download some books for holiday reading/listening, and keep up with email and Facebook. Hema decided she wanted to use the I-Pod for music, which was fine. I was glad it was being used by her. I spent a Monday morning just enjoying the I-Pad and downloading free apps. The picture clarity was wonderful. It was so clear and clean compared to my Dell laptop and Droid phone which, to me, were both grainy and dull. I found the name

"Retina Display" apt as it seemed designed to be very easy for the eyes to use. It was a pleasure to return to Apple products for me. I used a Mac computer many years ago then, for some reason, always had PC related products provided in the workplace. The I-Pad was easy to use and the "accessibility" options are impressive. I did not need voice-over at this point but the ability to change font sizes and to zoom using tap commands was a major upgrade from the first generation "Literati" e-reader I had used for a while. I played with the white writing/black background option and other accessibility features and settled on a 32 point font. It made some of the screen commands that are located at the edges of the screen a bit awkward sometimes, but I could read the text on screen very well. Bill and Kolby had told me that Apple products were better for low vision and blind people, and they were right. I told myself that when I was back on full pay in August I would get rid of the Droid and switch to an I-Phone whenever the next one (5) came out. I did not change phones immediately, but it felt empowering to strategize.

I noticed that I was much more patient while getting to know the I-Pad. It was a little frustrating as things sometimes disappeared inexplicably from the screen, especially while writing emails, and it was sometimes hard to figure out how to go back to the previous search, for example on You Tube, but it was genuinely fun to play with. I did not shout or curse in anger when something did not make sense. There were a couple of times I interrupted Hema's grading to tell her how something did not quite make sense. She let me struggle with it momentarily, so I would learn to figure it out for myself. She told me recently that she thought I had become a little lazy with technology, as I had two staff members to do everything for me for the eight years while I was department head. She was right. I would need to make more of an effort to do things on my own, and learn the new tricks I had been buffered from by my staff. I did not get frustrated quickly, and simply put the thing aside for another month as I might have earlier in the year. Somehow I was getting a handle on where my eyes were, and I was more confident in working through the learning process with the I-Pad. For contrast, my mind glanced back to some dark moments in the dead of winter when things were declining rapidly and we had no real grip on how the story would proceed. I remember clinging to a pillow some nights alone and saying over and over to myself, Oh no! Oh No! Oh No!, as my mind contemplated the horror of the rapid path to blindness that was a real possibility at that time. Those were terrible times. Now I found myself much more optimistic about my condition, and more positive in my reactions to things as a result.

One early summer day I even had a momentary fantasy about buying a motor cycle while watching an ad for a Honda 250 cc on television. This was a silly dream as I could not really ride one safely, it was just my minds way of telling me that I was feeling positive and confident about my vision. Perhaps it was also partly symptomatic of turning 50 which I would do in just a month from now—a sort of "mid-life moment" some might say. Either way, cruising to the coast on a motorcycle was a fun, if unrealistic, dream.

I also set about working more in the yard, and I enjoyed being outside even when the sun was bright. I always wore protective sunglasses and waited usually until after 4 pm each day to go out and work in the early summer sun. Despite yellow jacket stings, a spider bite, a long painful round with poison ivy, and the never ending primordial push of weeds and grass, the fruit growing on my trees, as well as the roses that were resurging for a second round of blooms, and the vegetables I had planted, all gave me much joy. For the first time in a long time I began to plan which stones I would cut for jewelry. I dusted and cleaned the ones I had cut over the years and savored looking at them and imagining them as pendants in jewelry. As my optimism and positivity were on the rise, so too was my level of activity and creativity. I wanted to be productive, much more than I had in a while. Because Hema had so much grading to do, we decided to postpone our trip to see Tim in Georgia. We stayed home and got lots done. In the middle of an activity I remembered that I had emailed my eye condition details to Suresh immediately after our DC trip and realized that I never heard back from his ophthalmologist wife. Perhaps he had many things to organize as he is relocating to India after retiring here in the US. They divorced soon after this, so my guess was, looking back, that she was already not taking much interest in his friends and their problems.

I was a little disappointed to find out that the books I needed to download to my I-Pad for my upcoming fall classes were not available on I-books. I was hoping I could have them on my I-Pad and use them in prepping for my classes and perhaps even use it in class. I remember that Bill and Kolby had advised me against this and now I know why. They were not even available, and clicking around with the device during class might not work well. I would have to rethink this need. I made a note to myself to contact disability services on campus (Later renamed The Office of Accessibility) to see if they might have a magnification device that I could borrow. I could have contacted my department head again but he said there was no money he could spare to buy me a desk for my new office, so I did not think there was much point in asking to have one bought for me through the department. I did not want to be pegged as the overly needy faculty member, always asking for something. I had gotten an I-Pad and a larger computer screen recently as accommodations, and then a resounding "no" to my request for furniture, so I figured I had already pushed my luck a little!

Being Handled, Muddling Through, and Owning the Narrative

I emailed the disability services director on campus, introduced myself, and briefly outlined my needs Tuesday May 11th. Only a day later, I got a very friendly email welcoming me back to campus from my research leave. Oddly, he apologized up front for being slow to respond, which he was not. Was I being "handled" I wondered—a genteel opening then nothing much to follow? The email stated that students in the same circumstances would normally be provided equipment through a state agency, and therefore—reading between the lines—I assumed not through the Office of Disability Services. He did not mention which agency or how faculty might be accommodated. Mmme, I am being pointed somewhere else I thought … The director said that they did not have portable equipment (to magnify my book or notes while teaching) but that I could come and use their facility in any way that might be useful. So I quickly gathered there was no provision for work related help through them—nothing I could use in my office or classroom, but lots of good will. I could come there and read books, and he was willing to meet to discuss other forms of "text access"—presumably meaning audio conversion, which I did not need at this point. I do think he was genuine in reaching out to offer help but they would not be able to provide what I needed. He suggested that I go through my department for help as a reading aid would be a "reasonable accommodation" under ADA. I was grateful for the advice (although I was being pointed somewhere else again), and I did not really expect them to have equipment sitting around that I could borrow. But, it seemed to me, there was a significant organizational gap here—a "blind spot" if you will. There was no one to talk to, or to coordinate support for me specifically as a faculty member.

I told Kolby about my contact with the ODS office, and she said she was not surprised they were not much help. She wanted to share something with me about what they said to her when she went to pick up the hard copies of the books she had given them to convert to audio. I would have to wait until later when we would get together to hear her experiences, but I could tell they were not going to be positive ones. She told me she was used to being her own advocate which I took to mean that there would not be much proactive help from others. I would need to learn how to be my own advocate, as she had been for herself. She had graduated with a 4.0 GPA, and is now busy in training to be a court reporter—all with no eye sight.

With this in mind, I immediately went online to look at equipment that might help me. CCTV units for magnifying books started at $2000 and up from there. I could not do it myself and my department had no money for such big purchases just for me and my specific needs. There were many other needs relating to core function of research and teaching that needed to be met. After talking it over with Hema, I decided to go through the Dean's office directly for any upcoming needs. She was a little concerned about bypassing my department head but I was more concerned about being able to get things done where there were more resources likely to be available, a little further up the organizational chart. I actually do not think he would have minded being bypassed on this one, equipment for low vision and blind needs was extremely expensive and departmental budgets were tight for now at least. Perhaps I could muddle through this first year back without any more major needs popping up. Perhaps I could find a simple magnifying device just to put over books that would suffice for now. I would try to take issues related to work one year at a time.

Looking back I thought that "muddling through" was a good term in capturing much about how the experience felt so far. I never once came across an easy path to information, advice, and advocacy. It felt much more like a process of making do, and of figuring out as we went along. Building incremental knowledge about my conditions, what to do, and how to adapt, became a central focus for Hema and me. Certainly there were good generic information sources online—lists of do's and don'ts to follow relating to eye health, and macular degeneration more specifically. Certainly my medical team members were excellent and caring. Certainly people in the workplace were well meaning. But I could not help but feel there was nothing really "certain" except that there were so many gaps and never a full and clear picture about any aspect of this condition. Perhaps such an idea was mythical and unrealistic—when did we ever really have this in life? Perhaps muddling through was how most of us lived, and also how people adapted to disability, we just were not aware of this consciously so much in everyday life. Ironically, even websites selling vision aids were often lacking in the simplest accommodations of design for their target audiences—low contrast color combinations, small lettering, difficult navigation directions, and so on, were common. I could not imagine how it would be for the poor souls who were out there trying to figure things out while dealing with more catastrophic or rapid vision loss than myself. For me I was "muddling" a lot but I was getting "through" things quite well. If the balance swung more towards muddling then things quickly slipped into the realm of "struggle." Kolby was right about the need to be one's own advocate, self-advocacy might be the only way to make sure I made it through the muddling. Although I would be muddling through much of the time, I also resolved to enjoy life as much as possible.

Somewhere in the spring, I just lost interest in wine and alcohol more generally. Something inside told me it was not a good thing for my eyes. Perhaps it was all of the hidden sugar in white wine that I knew was not good. Perhaps it was the fact that alcohol was a blood thinner which probably was counterproductive when treading carefully around bleeding and swelling blood vessels in the eyes. It is possible that it was some echo of a legend about homemade booze making people blind I was responding to unconsciously. Some websites listed wine as a positive, but I think only under the rubric that red wines contained good antioxidants, and perhaps the theory came from the wine industry itself. There were better ways to get those. I did not stop entirely, and the occasional glass of wine or single malt was nice, but it was becoming far from part of my regular routine. I tried to explain the change to a friend by saying that drugs and alcohol were ways that people escaped from or at least "enhanced" reality and that, when going through vision loss, your instinct is to try to *hold onto* reality as you know it. The last thing I wanted was for my grasp on reality to slip away, even momentarily.

In mid-June, Hema sent me a link to the exciting "Artificial Retina Project" (http://artificialretina.energy.gov/). Their home page includes the following information:

> "The U.S. Department of Energy's (DOE's) Artificial Retina Project is a collaborative, multi-institutional effort to develop an implantable microelectronic retinal prosthesis that restores useful vision to people blinded by retinal diseases. The ultimate goal of the project is to restore reading ability, facial recognition, and unaided mobility in people with retinitis pigmentosa and age-related macular degeneration. The project taps into the unique research technologies and resources developed at DOE national laboratories to surmount the many technical challenges involved with developing a safe, effective, and durable product. The research team includes six DOE national laboratories, four universities, and private industry."

This was exciting. Perhaps out of this and other collaborations, sometime in the future, people could be helped to see again. Hopefully, restoring vision would someday be a standard procedure, either through this implant, or through transplant technology. It was comforting but, my guess was, this was a long time into the future before it was readily available.

In late June Hema was busy finishing up summer school grading, and we were also preparing for our upcoming trip. This preparation largely consisted of getting together with people we would not see for a while and (mostly her) shopping for small gifts for friends and relatives we would see on the visits to England and India. I could not think of what to get my twin brother for our 50th we would celebrate together—a nice cardigan, perhaps. Hema, by contrast, had little trouble picking out things for the extended family she would buy gifts for. Her family and community ties back home were much stronger, and she would know just what to get each person. We made a list of what needed to be done before we got on the plane. I spent an hour or two on fair days getting the yard in shape to be gone for three weeks. We enjoyed picking the first figs and chili peppers of the summer, and I remembered back to last year not knowing if I would be able to see well enough to enjoy the garden this year at all. But it worked out well and things were in a good place. Happily the talk of eye problems was eclipsed by these activities. I even managed to avoid making an appointment for my routine eye exam until we would get back! I did set up my I-Pad so that I could continue writing notes on the trip but, otherwise, vision problems and their surrounding discourse were nicely in the background for a change.

I set up my new office on campus before we left. I moved in some furniture from home with the kind help of Steve and his truck. When we finished unpacking and I had arranged everything the next day, the room was relaxed and already familiar. I knew I would enjoy this space. The next afternoon the staff came over to see what I had done with my new office. I do not think they expected to see me there, but the tech support guy fit me in then to resurrect my computer which had been in storage for a year, so I met them there at short notice. The two staff members were trying to update me on an office drama for which I had no interest. I told them, only half-jokingly, to keep all of the negativity and drama in Ferguson building as here, in Curry, we were all about peace and love! They told me the story anyway, something about a missing office chair and a faculty tantrum. I had resolved upon my return to stay out of office politics, dramas, conflicts, and all things negative. I did not know how long I had with vision at my current level and I did not want to waste the time being caught up in trivia, or dragged into dramas, of which there was always a supply. Do not waste good and precious time on bad and pointless things—do *YOUR* thing, would become my work related mantra going into the new academic year. I wanted to write, teach and have fun just doing my thing—being *me* in a refreshingly different way. Eric, the tech support guy did an excellent job getting my old computer set up in the new space. The new "big screen" for my computer was very sharp and clear and not so huge that it looked ridiculous, or drew attention to my vision problems. I did not feel like I would need to explain the big screen when people visited, which was good.

I wanted to find a couple of Degas prints for my new office. He had suffered from a similar eye disease to me, and I found his resolve to be creative, and express his art in spite of these troubles, inspiring. I particularly liked his later work which relied less on details which he could not see, and more on impressions and on interior scenes. If outside, he painted at dusk or dawn when the light was not intolerably bright for him. He had become an impressionist by necessity not choice, as fine detail eluded him, and then he had become famous as a leader in the movement. It would be a good connection to my predecessors and a good way to begin conversation on the topic with people who might stop by my office and ask about the pictures. I settled on two pictures: "Peasant girls bathing in the sea at dusk" and "Dancers in Blue". Somehow both pictures spoke to me of his drive to communicate using his visual art, the joy he found in human movement and color—especially dance, and everyday activities like bathing, and the sorrow and bitter irony behind losing the sense most central to his chosen medium of capturing it—vision. Often I would look at the pictures and imagine him writing to his dear friend:

> "I see even worse this winter, I do not even read the newspapers a little; it is Zoé, my maid, who reads to me during lunch. Whereas you, in your rue Sadolet in your solitude, have the joy of having your eyes … Ah! Sight! Sight! Sight! … The difficulty of seeing makes me feel numb."—Edgar Degas, letter to friend, Evariste de Valernes, Paris, 6 July, 1891.

I felt for him.

· 9 ·

SEVENTH INJECTION

July 27th 2012

The seventh injection was on the same day as the opening ceremony at the London Olympics, and I was excited to watch it with Hema later that night. It was also two full months since I had been to the clinic, and had the last set of injections. I had not noticed any huge changes to my sight since last time so "injection day" was starting with good energy in the air. Hema was able to come with me to the retina clinic. I drove and she would drop me off, take the car to do some errands, and then pick me up when I was done. I was glad she was able to be there as it looked like it was going to be a very bright day, so being driven home would be a welcome blessing. On the way there, Hema questioned the route I took, which quickly made me annoyed. I thought she was starting to tell me there was a better, faster, way to the clinic. I told her that I came this way each time, and that it had the minimum turns and no need to cross traffic without a light on the way back. I remember adding "END OF STORY" to the end of my sentence. My speech surprised me at the time, as it did her, but it stopped the topic from developing and expanding, and making me more annoyed. Driving this way was my ritual born of need, and I did not want it questioned. She told me she was simply asking—trying to understand "why?" Momentarily I grew tense and slightly resentful—wishing I had simply come by myself. The moment passed, and we were soon at the clinic. Despite the tense moment, I was genuinely glad she was with me, and happy that she would pick me up around 11 am when I was likely to be done. I hated the fact that I got annoyed at small things, but I just wanted a peaceful journey there and back, and questioning my routine was not welcome.

The waiting room was quite full, so I estimated—given a 9:15 am appointment—that we would be done by between 11 and 11:30 am. Hema had some errands to run, so she left. I heard a middle aged African American woman behind me say to her mother, who was a patient, that she thought they kept us waiting for at least an hour so that the insurance would kick in and "they get they money" (sic). She apparently worked in a hospital, so she had some inside knowledge that we did not. They had been waiting for over an hour, and she was clearly annoyed that the appointment time never matched the treatment time. She had a fair and accurate point, but it was very rare to hear a critical comment in the waiting room. She was antsy to get moving and even complained to the staff. They simply told her that they would be called soon. Good for her, I thought. A lot of time is wasted just waiting around—*being patient*—and there is really not much you can do about it except bring something to do, or someone to talk to.

The eye test always felt like a failure for me. At first, even on the first test line for my (better) left eye, I could not see anything but big blotches of color in front of my eyes—predominantly blue but with other colors mixed in. I had not experienced this before and, for whatever reason, I did not say anything. After a few seconds there was the familiar clunk-clunk feeling of my eye as the line came closer into focus. I thought I had done badly, but I think the new technician simply started me off at a smaller line than usual, so I did not get the sense of momentum and achievement that comes with blazing through the bigger, easier, letter lines. I asked how I did compared to last time, and she told me I was slightly better in the left, and just slightly worse in the right—though neither at a significant level. I was happy to get through the retinal photos, again done by a new staff member. After the long initial wait, I was moving through the process quickly now.

Dr. Sanders came in to the room, and was quick to tell me that the images showed really good news—things were stable, and there was no need to continue the treatments beyond this final injection. He was thrilled and, then, so was I. I had many questions but held them off in order to simply go with the positive moment. Mirroring the last injection, he told me that things were as good as they would be at this point, and that the treatment had been successful. He added that he was really glad my vision had not "plummeted." This was the first time I had heard him use this word, and it was a really heavy one.

Perhaps he had saved it for when he knew it was not a reality. But, momentarily, this single word brought home the reality of where I could have been but was not. For the past year, I had been precariously balanced on the edge with a long drop—a plummet—into chaotic darkness just a step away into a parallel world that might have been.

The injection procedures passed quickly for me. When I was alone with the technician for a moment, she told me it was nice to see some people get good news. I said I guessed it was not always that way. She agreed, adding that they sometimes grow to really like patients and want the best for them, but not everyone gets the good news that treatment is over—even temporarily. I felt fortunate and, again, wanted to connect with others and to hear their stories of lives changed, lessons learned, and the importance of talk and relationships. I told Dr. Sanders I would still like to conduct some interviews with patients and he was still enthusiastic. We would sit down with a coffee at some point soon he said. As he left the room he added, "Doesn't that sound nice … to sit down with a cup of coffee?!" He was off to the next patient and then on call for the weekend, dealing with whatever misfortune befalls others worse off than me. We never did collaborate on research, or even have coffee, but it was the start of some important ideas for me.

Savoring Life

As usual, upon my return home, Hema had lovely food ready. I ate and fell asleep for two hours as I always did. I felt good, and the steely intrusion into my eye did not have many side effects this time. We relaxed that evening and watched the opening ceremony rerun on NBC. I was proud of the show—highlighting British culture and history, as linear and modern a historical account as it was. But my eyes lost their zest for this day half way through the less spectacular parade of nations. These athletes had so much drive, so much passion, and so much hope focused on the next couple of weeks. I felt like I had been given a reprieve—good news when others got bad news. Stability when others were experiencing plummeting loss. How would I use the good time I had been given? I was no Olympian, but I found the life force of these athletes and competitors inspiring and message-full—*get on with what you need to get on with while you're in the moment where you can.*

The next day I reveled in going through the photographs from the recent travels and sent some out to people. I picked peppers from the garden, and enjoyed touching the cantaloupes that had appeared while we were gone. They felt like sweet warm babies heads in my hand. A few had turned orange in the warm sun and had dropped off the vines as if to announce they were ready to eat, and they were. It was a joy to be home and to not be in constant motion as we had been on our travels, and to see things so alive and fruitful here. I went to pick up my guitar from Arts house where he had kept it safely while we were out of the country. I played with the rocks I had picked up on Filey beach—imagining how I might cut them, and we watched the early events from the Olympics.

I craved some time just to be alone and enjoy being in the moment but I also loved having Hema around. She also loved being around but hated driving back and forth to her apartment all the time. We were adjusting back to life here after being gone for a few weeks and in constant motion, and constant contact with others. Things had been busy with travel and would be busy again soon when the new academic year began in August. Now was the time just to enjoy the small things in the space between bigger things, as much as we could.

After being around family so much, it seemed natural for us to talk more about our own move towards marriage. We had no specific date or plan at this point. I knew Hema wanted to move to a bigger house where family could come and visit for extended periods, so we started looking at houses. We did not have the funds to make the transition at this point, but it was fun to drive around neighborhoods where I would be comfortably close to food sources, and where she felt good about living and having family visit. The bigness of the upcoming semester and new academic year loomed quickly, and the house hunting slipped from our activities for a while. We needed to save money before we could move anyway.

Back to School After a Year's Leave

Just before the semester started in August my workout pal, Jon, returned from Brazil where he spends summer breaks (their winters) with his Brazilian wife. She lived and worked there. He emailed to tell me he would not be there on the first day back, and to ask me how I was doing. He joked that if I did not respond to the email he would know my eyes had taken a dramatic turn for the worse, so much so that I could not see or respond to emails! It was a fun way to make sure I responded, and why not learn to build and accept—perhaps invite—humor into the vision-loss journey?

When I returned to the first faculty gatherings, no one asked me what I had been working on during my research leave so, at first, I did not introduce the topic of my experience with vision loss. A few people knew but I did not tell everyone. I was not quite sure how to articulate how my impairment would affect them, other than that I might not recognize them from a distance. So I held off on this. Besides, everyone was busy establishing themselves into the new academic year, and were focused on their own news and goals. This was fine as it meant I did not have to discuss it publicly if asked. But I have to admit I was a little disappointed in the lack of collegial interest in what I had been doing while away for a whole year. It was a chilly reception from people for whom I had advocated for eight years. But it was time to get on with my own story.

I was ready for my new classes starting Monday August 20th at 2 pm. I sat in my new office and at 1:50, and slightly nervous, I told myself it is time to go meet the class and start this new chapter of my career as a regular faculty member. Lots of newness! I walked into the classroom and up front was another professor. She told me this was Spanish, and then a number I do not recall. "AHHH my class must have been moved," I thought to myself. I panicked slightly, wondering where it might be. I tried the next room, I do not know why because it is unlikely to be the next room. If it had been moved, it was more likely to a different building. It was not the class next door. "Oh no," I thought, "what a start"! I rushed back to my office and searched on the schedule system for my class. It was listed as 2 pm on Tuesday/Thursday. I had the wrong day! In over fifteen years here I had never made this mistake. I looked back at the schedule draft sent out months earlier and, sure enough, it was listed as Tuesday/Thursday. I had missed the visual detail and, in my mind, convinced myself that it was Monday/Wednesday. I had requested this in order to spread out my teaching over four days. I had not done a full teaching load in nine years, so I knew I needed to spread out the work and the energy and preparation time it would demand. I went to my department head's office and he said he did not remember hearing from me to correct the Tuesday/Thursday as listed on the schedule draft, then deflected me off into another topic—new pictures from his family summer trip he had put up on his wall. I was stressed out at the thought of all of my classes being on two days, but he was not conscious of my worries, so I made small talk for a minute then left, disappointed. This, after the trash I had been given for furniture, and I was beginning to wonder if I was welcome back here. I was being overly sensitive. I went back to my office and looked through emails. I had not corrected the mistake, but did find my original request which was for Monday/Wednesday for this class and Tuesday/Thursday for the other two. I decided to drop the issue. Nothing could be done at this point anyway. A couple of days later I heard from my department head. He had also gone back through emails and not found a correction request, so I emailed him my original request and suggested something went wrong in developing the draft of the schedule, but that I should have caught it on the draft. I was trying to share responsibility for the slip-up, but I never heard back from him on the topic. He let me to take the blame. The important point is, I had missed a detail I never would have missed before my eyes declined, and it annoyed me. But I regrouped, and tried to convince myself that teaching just on two days might be a blessing in disguise. It actually worked out fine, once I got used to the enormous energy required on Tuesdays and Thursdays.

The first week of classes was a blur of activity. Positive energy abounded, and it felt good to be back in the classroom talking about things that interested me. I made sure my lecture notes were large print and that I knew more or less what I was going to say by memory so that I did not have to read much in front of the class. To have a blur-out trying to read notes would have been embarrassing. I had printed their names on the roll list in large font also. I could see their faces quite well, even at the back of my classrooms, and I think all went quite smoothly. I did not tell them anything about my visual impairment because, at first, I was not sure how it would affect things. After the first week I thought that I should be alright without telling them. I wanted to play it by ear and see if we would need any strategic accommodations on either of our parts. Besides having one or two blurry moments talking to students after class, I was fine. My blood pressure was probably elevated from teaching, and I did have a few moments where faces, even close-up, were hard to see clearly.

While working out at the gym one early morning during that first week of classes, a retired guy—Chris—who works out regularly, came over to introduce himself as a fellow macular degeneration patient. Jon had told him that I too had this disease, and I was glad he had. He was the first person I had met (that I know of) who was going through the same treatment I had been through. His left eye had the tell-tale signs of post injection redness, which is what tipped off Jon. Although I already knew him well enough to say hi to, he came over and shook my hand as if to meet again, this time as a fellow sufferer of a similar disease. He shared with me that he had been through three injections so far. I told him I had had seven. We chatted briefly and he was relatively upbeat and matter of fact about it, even downplaying the injection experience, but I thought that I would invite him at some point to chat more about it. He did say he had a cousin who had the same thing, so they suspected a genetic component in his case. We even joked about the treatment a little—mimicking the macabre moment when they clip your eyes open, and the needle comes unavoidably towards you! It was fun and meaningful to share this with him.

Losing Bud

On Friday evening at the end of the first exhausting week of classes for both Hema and me, I offered to take her out to dinner to Phoenix which was one of her favorite restaurants. We sat outside, and enjoyed a nice dinner in the late summer evening. It had been a long hard week. It was the first week of teaching for me in a year, and the first week of an incredibly busy semester of teaching seven classes for Hema. We enjoyed the low-humid evening. As we sat there, I received a Facebook message from a dear friend: Christine Keisinger. This was a little unusual as we did not talk that often, and we had just touched base a day or two before. I did not open it, but figured it had something to do with our mutual friend, Bud Goodall, who had been sick from an infection. A bug must have caught him weak from his chemo and radiation and all of the related medications he had cheerfully embraced in what he called his "Adventures in Cancerland."

After dinner we went to Target to shop for some specific items. I dropped Hema off back at her car outside the restaurant. She was going to her place to finish some work, so I drove home alone. The evening was getting dark and I could tell the long, light, summer nights were just waning and starting to get a little darker a little sooner. I dreaded the upcoming morning and evening darkness of winter, and the glare of oncoming headlights once again, but it had been a good week and all was looking good for a nice weekend. As I was driving along the very familiar battleground avenue towards home, I must have been daydreaming because I lost track of where I was. I looked around, wishing I could find a visual clue. Panic rose quickly in me. "OH MY GOD, WHERE AM I? *WHERE AM I?*" I spoke loudly into the dimming twilight. For a few seconds *I had no idea where I was*. I knew I was in Greensboro, but it all sort of looked the same unless something stood out, and at that moment nothing did. Somehow my brain backtracked and told me that I was driving home from New Garden Road towards home, so I must be on Battleground Avenue. But, for a brief moment, nothing I could see was telling me exactly where I was. It was a terrifying feeling. As I finally sat back and relaxed, I began to recognize landmarks. Lowe's on the right, and the double turn lane to the left onto Pisgah Church Road. "Ahhh!"... I thought ... "The relief of the familiar," but it added to my dread of the nights that were inevitably drawing in towards fall and winter. I would have to teach myself while driving alone in the dark to be mindful of where I was, and perhaps even speak out my location loudly and regularly so that I did not lose track of my whereabouts. I immediately adopted this strategy. A few nights later I tried it and it helped a lot ... "Ok you're on Battleground coming home from music night at Steve's ... you're coming up to the light at Westridge. There's your bank on the right. There's Applebee's on the left. Now the left at Pisgah Church Road ..." The sections that had fewest noticeable landmarks would be where I would talk to myself the most so I did not lose where I was.

When I got home I checked my I-Pad to find that Christine was emailing me to say she just saw announced on Facebook that Bud had died. I was shocked but not terribly surprised. His wife had announced a day or two before that he had an infection, and they had called hospice, "just in case." I was deeply saddened by the loss of a dear friend and amazing scholar and person. People were making very touching statements on his wall that had been kept going for that purpose. I wanted to wait to think about what to say. That night I felt the loss of a dear friend and constant supporter in this journey so far. Just days before, we had talked about us coming out to see him when the weather got cooler in Arizona, and suddenly he was gone. Gracefully, he always talked as if we had parallel journeys, but his was much more finite than mine. He never pointed this out as we simply supported each other. The next morning I wrote on his wall, "I will miss you my dear friend. I find comfort in knowing that your soul delights in new mysteries ... You always loved a good mystery! XOXO"

I would miss his genuinely positive communication in the form of advice, encouragement, and the connections between our experiences and stories we created as he held onto life, and I held onto my sight. He was a major source of support for me as well as an old and close friend. We had shared many mystery novels back and forth over the years, and he wrote at length about mystery, hence the reference in my post to "mystery." Looking back at our last email exchange before he died he was glad we were making plans to visit, and he closed our Facebook chat with:-) ... So much can be said with a simple smile.

Early on Wednesday at the gym, I kidded with Chris—asking if he was using his eye drops, and he said yes. He shared that during the last injection he could actually see bubbles in his eye, something I never experienced. I asked him if he had seen the halo shape that I had many times, and he said no. He asked me if my "outlook" had improved now that things had stabilized and I told him yes, definitely. Was he telling me he was frightened or depressed I wondered? He was acting quite matter of fact about it, but you never know. I joked that people's faces were less distorted, which was good, but the downside was that I could now see my own gray hairs more clearly! We laughed and left it at that, returning to our respective workouts.

A Family/Genetic Connection?

In late August, my dad informed me that my uncle who, at the time of the call in late August 2012, was 83 was undergoing tests after complaining of some of the same things I have experienced. Perhaps there is a genetic link for me after all? Perhaps it's more about being 83 for him, but it was certainly an interesting coincidence. I made a note to find out more when he had been through the tests.

On the Thursday of my second week of teaching I stood in front of the second class of the day. I had just closed the windows that someone kept opening in the fresh early morning. By 11 am warm air was coming in, and the cool air conditioned air was seeping outside to no effect. After this, I pulled out my attendance roll sheet. I looked at the first name at the top of the list and I could not see the name clearly enough to announce it—to question if the person was present. "Oh no," "I thought", to myself … "please not a fuzz-out in front of the class." I stood there for a second or two with nothing happening, waiting and hoping for my eyes to focus. This few seconds was a long silence in front of a live audience. A few students clearly began to wonder what was happening. I became anxious and began to sweat in the clammy room. I stopped and told the class that I was visually-impaired and that my eyes sometimes took a few seconds to focus. Some smiled or chuckled thinking I was joking. I did not know how to tell them I was not joking, but I let the moment go. After a few seconds I could see again, so I moved ahead with the humdrum task of taking attendance. Later, I wondered how kind students would be to an instructor who was disabled—specifically blind. Part of me believed that many of them would be understanding and sensitive, and part of me though that many of them probably would not be.

On the Sunday of Labor day weekend I decided to cut a stone for the first time in months. I had a small piece of petrified palm wood—a stone I have always liked—ready to cut. I sailed through the process and put on my magnification glasses at the end, just to make sure I had done a perfect job.

My heart sank. I had missed a couple of rough spots on the all-important edges of the stone. How could I have rushed through just assuming it was fine, I asked myself? I cursed, recognizing that I had been overly confident, and not systematic enough in checking my work along the way. I would have to go back and start again, carefully making sure that all the flat and rough spots that would detract from the smooth curved polish necessary for a finished stone, were eliminated. I just wasted an hour by not being methodical in checking my work at each stage—something I never had to do when my eyes were in good shape. Perhaps these small reminders to be more thorough and deliberate would keep me from making bigger mistakes where they might really count.

In an odd twist of timing, on that Labor-day weekend I got an email from my twin brother, David, in response to my inquiry about his recent test results from a liver scan. It went as follows:

David:	"All is clear, so nothing to worry about … But I am having some problems with my eyes so have a scan on 17 Sep—will let you know. Otherwise ok."
Me:	"Ok well the results are good. What problems with the eyes specifically?"
David:	"Takes a while to focus and bring text into focus-especially left eye."
Me:	"Hopefully it's just normal aging. But it is one of the symptoms I have. It will help your ophthalmologist to know I have Cone Dystrophy and wet macular degeneration. They can look for those. An optometrist won't have the same diagnostic technology."

A day later he popped back with, "Ok. Yes thanks, will do, hawk-eye!"

Waiting for the eyes to focus is one of the symptoms I have experienced quite regularly, most recently in front of a class of students. So I know how this creates difficulties. With my uncle on my father's side also experiencing similar issues, perhaps a part of the bigger picture itself was struggling to come into focus. They both had tests scheduled, and I would be following them closely for connections that would help us all make sense of what was happening with our eyes. Luckily he was not experiencing other symptoms, or at least he was not aware of them yet. But, as much as the bigger picture emerging was interesting and potentially illuminating, I had a bad feeling about this. It was unlikely to be normal aging as I had optimistically framed my email, but there was hope that it could be, and he has been through so many health battles that he really did not need another one. I noticed his emails did not engage with my experiences and diseases at all. I could tell he was hoping he did not have what I had, so I filled in the information as if he had asked. He could look up the conditions for himself if he wanted to, or put off thinking about it until the test day rolled around. I assumed he would choose the latter. Either way, I would have to wait a few weeks for their results and another piece of the puzzle to emerge. I told Hema his symptom, and she said, "That's a little scary for me." I agreed. Eye problems are a little scary. I let the new nickname "Hawkeye" slide without comment, ascribing it to the acidity of "British humor"!

As much running around as Hema did in her old Nissan Sentra, it was time to think about getting her a newer car, but she did not quite see it that way. She insisted that it was me who needed a new car—one that was set higher up, an SUV for example, but I was not convinced that I would ever need a new car. She saw this as pessimism. I would have been happier buying her a newer car that was small enough for her to drive comfortably. Her thinking was that I needed a car that was higher up to help me see, and she could drive my old car. But I liked my old car, and it was too big for her. When driving mine, she had to sit on a cushion to see the road, and then push the seat all the way forward, as the pedals were a long way away. She was too close to the steering wheel and the air bag. Besides, the issue was not me being able to see up and over things, but rather being able to see well enough at all. So why not get her a car and I keep mine until I could no longer legally drive? If I was driving for a while, a few years for example, then I would keep it for a while. If I could not drive much longer, then we would get rid of my car and use her newer one for both of us, with her as the driver. Her perspective seemed perfectly logical to her, and mine did to me, but no one was willing to go with the other's perspective. So nothing happened. We were at friendly impasse on the subject. We were both still driving our own old cars well into the fall semester, and would probably be doing so until hers just stopped working, or until I made a firm decision to do something specific.

Another Eye Exam

I finally made an appointment for a regular eye exam at Oman Eye Care for Wednesday 12th September. I would be going back to the place where this story essentially began over a year ago, when Dr. Johnson noticed some odd patterns on my retinas and insisted on me going to see Dr. Sanders. I would fill her in on the story since then, and would make a point of thanking her for their diligence in sending me to Dr. Sanders, as it helped me get essential treatment early.

At the eye exam I went through the usual miserable struggles with the letter tests. The nurse told me that nobody likes them, even people with good vision. I hated these tests. These days they always felt like failure. The first screen came up and she asked me how far down the lines I could read. I told her I could not read any of them! At other moments I guessed at the letters based on a slight curve or a line that went a certain way that suggested a letter might be more likely. However, I could not see very many of them clearly at all during the test. Nor could I specifically distinguish an H versus an M, and F versus a P, or an O versus a D, for example. It was depressing and stressful. We even had to stop to wipe the tiny lenses in front of me because I was steaming them up from my stress level.

We worked our way through the detailed vision tests, "… Is it clearer with a, or b …? Which one is clearer now c, or d?" none of them looked particularly clear. This produced a diagnosis of 20/50 in the left and 20/70 in the right, where I knew I had significant damage since the last visit. Much had happened in my eyes in the year since Dr. Johnson, my Optometrist, saw me. She asked me how I was adjusting and I told her about some everyday activities such as reading. We talked about the joys of the I-Pad, and then we talked about driving. This was the part that I dreaded. I was not going to mention it, but she asked. I told her that I already restricted myself to places with which I was familiar, and limited my night driving when it was dark to roads that had a median, and avoided unfamiliar interstates where I typically had a hard time reading signs. She told me that I would fail the driving test, but that she was pleased that I already restricted my driving, as the DMV would likely give me a restricted license closely paralleling what I already did. She clarified that I would be legal to continue driving if my eyes did not deteriorate much more, but that I would be restricted to ensure everyone's safety. Good news—bad news, I know, but it was better than I had feared. I had imagined that they would tell me I should not be driving at all. Doctor Johnson put it aptly when she said that losing the privilege to drive is a massive shift in people's sense of independence. I agreed. This potential loss had played on my mind significantly before going into the appointment. I had almost put off going for another year, but I knew I had to face where I was and what that meant.

I told her about my twin brother's upcoming appointment, and her eyes grew wide with interest at the possible genetic factor. None of us knew the origins of the Cone Dystrophy, or the connection between the Cone Dystrophy and the wet macular degeneration. His complaint of eye problems might be an unfortunate but tantalizing piece of the causal puzzle. She went on to suggest that if it turned out to be just signs of aging in his eyes, then environmental factors that were different in my life might have exacerbated the genetic factors we both shared somewhere in our DNA. I half joked that my living in the sunnier climate of the US, and he in gloomier England, might be that factor, and it actually could be.

I asked her about the frequency of cases she sees of Cone Dystrophy and, as I thought, these were rare. Macular degeneration sufferers were much more common especially, she had found, in people with light colored eyes, or who had worked outside much of their lives, or who smoked, or who had high blood pressure, and a family history of the disease. Her experience matched that of the research I had found months ago. As for me, I suspected there was a genetic predisposition that was compounded by having blue eyes and inadequate eye protection while outside for activities my whole life. Whether true or not, it seemed like a plausible working narrative of how things might fit together.

The assistant walked me to the front desk and said she noticed some slight scratches on my lenses, and asked if I wanted to look at some new glasses today. I said no thanks, and that I would come back another day. As I left, I was thinking to myself that slightly scratched lenses were the least of my worries, but I did not say anything. She was just doing her job, trying to get me into the area where I might try on and purchase new glasses. I imagined that the mark-up on glasses was substantial given what they were.

I drove the short distance home in the bright light and rested for an hour while the dilation lessened enough for me to look at the computer screen. I made a strong cup of tea and sat down to begin work. Hema called from her campus and I explained the driving situation as well as my worsening prescription since last year. When I told her I would fail the driving test because of my vision, she was struck by the gravity of that, and said, "Really?" I told her I had been trying to tell her this for a while, and she said she had listened to me as I have been telling her. From then on in the phone call she just listened to my report from the appointment, and then we had to cut short the call because she bumped into her department head on campus. We would process the information more, later that day. I checked on line at the definition of "visually impaired" and most web sites specified 20/60 vision was the point of entry into that category. I was right there.

A New Car and a New Journey

Soon after the results from my regular eye test, Hema and I began to discuss what we would do about new cars again. This time I think Hema realized that I would not be doing much driving, so it made sense for me to keep my old, but reliable, and low mileage car, and for us to think about getting something newer for her. She was nervous about the purchase, but she drove a lot more than me, and her current car was very near death. We agreed to move this plan forward when we had a little time at fall break in a few weeks. I asked her not to block out that time with too many other errands or social events, as we would need time to look at cars and make the purchase. She agreed.

On September 17th I got a message from my twin brother after his retina scan appointment, and I quickly opened it in anticipation: "Had the scan today. There is a hole in each retina. Will send me to Moorfield's eye hospital for further checks. Will keep you posted."

I was stunned, but not entirely surprised, given his symptoms. But "holes"? I wasn't quite sure what he meant by holes. Were they the same dark circles I had from the Cone Dystrophy—dark circles that looked like holes, or were they tears in the retina—literally holes? Were his problems also in the macula or something different? I shot back with more questions and waited impatiently for some clarification.

A while later he popped back up and said: "I'm afraid the Dr. was not exactly communicative. He showed me the scans and the retina from the side view just dipped down in one place. He said it was a 'hole' but it just looked like the retina was a bit thinner in that place. Was that different from what you had?"

I went on to explain how my symptoms started and then ended with: "… Hopefully the specialist at the hospital will know what it is and have a name for it."

He was beginning the journey into finding out what was going wrong with his eyes, and it appeared that the first Doctor he saw was not particularly helpful or detailed, or just did not know what to name it. I was fortunate to get good help quickly and I hoped he would too, particularly if he had something degenerative. I wanted to be there for him in processing this problem. I did not know how to be involved for him during his two tough rounds with cancer years before. I just did not know what to do or say, but now I could empathize and perhaps anticipate what his questions and fears might be. A day later he popped back on Facebook again: "Ok thanks, will keep you posted."

At the end of September one morning at the gym, Chris approached me and said, "Well if it makes you feel any better I have to start injection in the other eye too!"

"Oh no" I replied.

"Yeah!" He added, pointing to the right eye.

"So that one started with the same thing", I asked. "When does that start … Will they stagger them like two weeks apart alternating … what's the deal?"

"I don't know I just go when they tell me to!"

"Wow, I am sorry to hear about that."

"Yeah I went in just for a follow up, and didn't think I would be getting an injection, and they told me then."

"Oh no, so you had one yesterday? And more to come."

"Well, we'll just keep at it" he added philosophically, "But my eyesight is getting better!" He added, hopefully, and adding an upbeat at the end of the brief but heavy account.

From here he quickly turned to commenting on my work out partner, Art's, Texas Longhorns shirt. He was looking for a humorous way out of the dark conversation. He talked about how their current coach left UNC to go there, and offended a lot of people in North Carolina. Despite the humor, he was about to start living through one of the great fears of those of us who have primarily one eye attacked. Namely, he was about to possibly lose his reliance physically and psychologically on having "one good eye." Being able to tell yourself … "yes but, I still have one good eye …" was a narrative lifeline to normality that would be hard to see slip away into the blurry darkness. The narrative corner this backs you into is much harder to deal with. He wanted to tell me, but I could tell he also wanted to stay light and positive about what was happening. I asked him about his blood pressure and he told me that he had been working on it for a long time, and that he was *just* in the normal range. The moment broke up quickly as we all moved in different directions for our respective next exercises. I know he was only trying to joke, but why would he even joke about his misfortune possibly making me feel better?

Future Plans and a Family Narrative Emerges

Seemingly out of the blue, once we were well into the busy swing of the new semester, Hema picked back up on the topic of having children. She said that she understood if we would not plan to have children. This opened up a good conversation about long term life plans between us. I said I thought she would make a wonderful mother, and she would, but that we were coming together in our lives at a point when having children would be difficult in terms of the energy needed, and the financial burden. I told her I would like us to be able to retire at a good age when we could still enjoy our lives, and travel together. If we had a child starting at fifty for me and almost forty for her, then that would be the defining thing in our lives from then on. I did not want to leave her behind when I died without many assets, and a child still in high school or college. I know she was torn on the subject, but I think that knowing how much energy it took to manage two busy careers helped us both understand how much more difficult it would be to start having children at this point in life. Behind the story was also my worry about my vision and having a family with the chance of me being disabled, and possibly passing it on to the child. We did not raise this issue explicitly in this conversation, although it was part of the backdrop to my reluctance to try to have children.

One day in September our friends from Raleigh, Venkat and Vidya visited. At their request, we took them to play par three golf. It was fuzzy and unclear but I could see my ball well enough to hit it reasonably well and find it on the course, and it was a fun adventure. I had not played since my eye problems started, and it felt good to go out and play as if all was well. Hema enjoyed playing so much that she went again alone a week or so later to practice. I wanted to be part of fulfilling her desire to play golf and tennis, so I made a note to myself to try to work in more of this during the fall, and before winter set in. I had no idea how tennis would work out visually for me, but I needed to give it a try for her. I remembered back to a documentary I saw a while ago in which a group of fully blind cricketers in India had developed a form of cricket for blind people. They found a way to play and enjoy participating by having a ball that made a noise, so it could be located by them while batting and fielding. So I could try tennis and golf for Hema's sake too.

Early one Thursday morning I was reaching around in my sock drawer for a pair of black socks to wear for work. I reached up with the other hand to turn on the lamp on top of the chest of drawers. I was not looking as I reached up. Clumsily I knocked over the stuffed bear Hema got me for Valentine's Day last year. In turn, the bear knocked over the small porcelain hand bell that Mum had given Hema as a token gift to remember her by. It fell behind the chest of drawers onto the hardwood floor with a light thud. My heart sank and I felt like an idiot for not being more careful. This object meant a lot to Hema and I had clumsily knocked it over and, as I suspected, it had broken. Thankfully it did not shatter, but the handle broke off. I left it right where it fell until after work because I did not want to see what I had done. I did not want to get any more annoyed with myself than I already was. When I retrieved it that evening I tried to see if it would glue back in reasonable condition. It might, but the crack would be obvious. I did not confess the accident to Hema until sometime later, but I did take the other object mum and dad had given us—a small porcelain vase—to Hema's apartment where it would be safer, and where she could enjoy it without the chance of me breaking that too. When I finally confessed weeks later she simply said, "No comment." That's all that was said on the topic.

In the beginning of October Hema's sister and her husband were having logistical complication relating to the child care of their daughter Sagarika while they were both at work. His parents used to watch her until her Mother got home. This arrangement was lost when his father got very sick, and was having treatment in a different city. They were no longer able to fulfill this duty as they had for a while. How to handle it was a complicated and difficult decision for them, and it was causing some conflict and strife between them. Should she give up her job, or should they hire someone for the childcare duties. Hema offered to help in any way we could. Rika was her God daughter and she wanted to fulfill this role (as well as being a good sister). She wanted to make a difference for the children in her life, and I knew partly she was working through the decision we were making about whether we would have children or not. If we were not having children ourselves, she would be the best Aunty and God mother she could be.

One Saturday morning we were walking in the park and chatting with mum and dad—our weekly phone call. I asked if David had an appointment set up yet, and Dad said he was still waiting to be notified by the hospital. I said I would drop him a note to see how that process was going and to emphasize the need for quick treatment if he could impact that in any way. He asked me how my eyes were doing, and if I had noticed any more decline since the last injection. I told him I could not really tell. He then asked me how driving was going. I told him I was careful and that I was more or less on a restricted driving plan. He asked if my eyes would come back to normal now that they were stabilizing. I told him again that no, I had irreversible damage and that there is no recovery of eye sight as such. There is no way back unless someone invents a way back. Again, he told me that I could have one of his eyes. I could feel the kindness in his words across the miles. Oddly that gray cool fall morning, the weather was the same here as it was where they were, temperature and all. Later that day I thought of a humorous response to his offer: If he was going to give me one of his eyes, and might need to give David one, then he would be in serious trouble himself! He would have liked the joke, I think, but better in the moment to let him express his selfless fatherly love.

In mid-October the luminous pattern I sometimes see when I close my eyes came back vividly. One night, as I closed my eyes to go to sleep, it appeared as if before me as a gray mass of varying shades, from light to dark. It quickly morphed from a gray mass to two interconnected heart shapes, to a three leafed clover, to a fallen oak leaf, and finally to a shape that looked like a US state, maybe Virginia or New York. My eyes were transfixed to the image as it seemed to cross my field of vision from left to right, while changing the whole time. Before it faded it looked like two or three large bright luminescent hairs on a camera lens surrounded by a cool gray comet like glow. Was this the medication working or the damaged area, expressing itself somehow as visual feedback? Perhaps the bright hair-like images were my own retinal veins I could see? I did not know what any of it really was, or what it meant, but every time it appeared it was fascinating to watch. Later it struck me how my mind locked onto and followed these images so intently, and then interpreted them somewhat within the context of what was going on at the time. For example, I had just been for a walk among the first fallen leaves of autumn at the park, and recently saw a program about comets. We had been talking about marriage and wedding plans which might include a trip to Niagara Falls, New York, as we walked in the beauty of fall. These recent experiences had to be a factor in how my brain interpreted what it thought my eyes were "seeing."

On my weekly call home on Sunday October 14th dad had an update for me on my Uncle Ernest's appointment. He had been for tests through the NHS. The doctor gave him the usual letter tests and looked closely into his right eye. Apparently the doctor had paused to announce, dramatically to him, that she could find nothing wrong with his right eye. He looked at her and, without missing a beat, announced right back that this made complete sense given that he had come to have his LEFT eye examined! Smartly, he took this as a sign that he should pursue treatment through private medicine, which he immediately did. He was pleased with the results and really liked his new doctor. They quickly administered several laser treatments to stop the retinal edema caused by blood vessel distortions. He did not have the exact condition that I had, but perhaps there was a familial connection nonetheless. Whatever the connection, we were both restricted to local driving and other common blurry struggles—him in a small picturesque village in Rutland, England, and me here in North Carolina.

My brother was having worse luck with the NHS. I had pushed him to call and find out when he would get an appointment at the famous Moorfield's in London where he had been referred. He wrote back to announce that they told him "18 Feb next year!" This would be over four months from the original trip to his primary care physician. He went on to say, "The waiting list is insane. But it's the national center (Moorfield's). There has to be a better way!" I hoped he would get quicker attention than this but, again, there too it seemed that other perhaps more critical and life threatening conditions took priority over eyes and vision loss.

I went on to tell him that if he noticed any signs of quick decline he should switch immediately to private medicine—even though it would be expensive. It was his call—wait, spend nothing, and hope for the best, or spend a lot of money but get immediate treatment and maybe head off a period of decline. But I was worried about how long it would be before he would even have a diagnostic appointment. A wait of four months was unbelievably long. I gave him some simple steps to help detect and monitor any signs of distortion or decline, and the topic closed there for a while. I held off on telling David that, depending on the condition he had, there was a chance that he could have passed it onto at least one of his three children. What good would that have done at that moment when he did not even have a clear story on what he had?

· 10 ·

THREE MONTH FOLLOW-UP

October 26th 2012

(Scene: **Waiting room**)

Patient's daughter:	"Well, I don't know if I can get him here then. I start chemo myself sometime around then, and so I am not sure exactly … (Pause)"
Claire:	"OK … (Pause) …"
Patient's daughter:	"Well, put him down for then and I will see what I can do"
Claire:	"OK we will see you then. Have a nice weekend …" She added warmly, but without engaging with the woman's complexity.

My heart went out to these people. This was a small but telling part of a conversation I overheard of a middle-aged woman (probably the daughter), making an appointment for a man (probably her father) who was well into his 70s, to come back for his injection four weeks from now. This would be right around thanksgiving. He stood to the side as she made arrangements. Given the four week interval, he was obviously deep in the throes of the treatment I had just been through. Clearly also, this was a family in which illness and health care had taken on an organizing centrality. They looked and sounded like blue-collar country folks, and I could only imagine their deepening struggle. I was sitting near the check-out counter close to the rooms where I would see Dr. Sanders for my three month check-up. Everything looked pink after the retina pictures, but until I met with him to go over the test results, I was not sure how rosy the pink really was.

It was a lovely cool, heavily overcast, gray, fall Friday, at the end of a busy week. It was a week packed with grading papers, which left my eyes exhausted. Just the very outer edges of incoming storm Sandy were bringing heavy cloud cover that would be good for me to drive home in after the appointment while still dilated. It would prove tragic for many when it came ashore the next day and beyond, but I had no idea just how deep and extensive a tragedy it would be as I enjoyed the cloud cover today. I checked in at the front desk as usual, paid the copay (which had gone up by $10 since my last visit, without explanation) and waited. The waiting room was sparsely populated today, so I knew I would probably be examined quite quickly. The eye test was conducted by George, a very small man with awkward bent legs. I did not know his condition, possibly CP, but I was impressed that the office had made a point of hiring someone with a physical disability. He ran me through the dreaded eye tests, then dripped the awful stinging dilation drops into my eyes, then he examined each eye through the microscope. He asked me if anything had changed, and I told him I could not detect any specific decline. I was very nervous when he announced that he would need a second opinion on the microscope test. I wondered what he had seen. Was this another area of bleeding, swelling? "Ugggh" I thought to myself worriedly, "what am I in for this time?" I stared forward and just waited for the moment to unfold. Just off to my side, they discussed the segment of the eye where he was pinpointing and documenting something, and I guessed from their conversation that she was perhaps still training him in this diagnostic test. I relaxed a little as she calmly encouraged me.

As the father and daughter whom I had overheard earlier left the office, my name was called to go into one of the consulting rooms. Sitting there waiting with the lights dimmed, I watched the familiar nature images on the monitors. These were interspersed with images of tropical beaches. A grass roofed hut stood invitingly in the warm bright sun on the edge of a point overlooking the crystal clear ocean somewhere. It was beautiful, but I could not imagine Hema and me sitting around in that bright sun—it was not our thing at all. On that we agreed completely, albeit for different reasons. As I inserted myself into these inviting images to pass the time, Dr. Sanders walked in with a warm greeting and a handshake. It was good to see him, although I had not missed being here for the past three months.

"Hi Mr. Kellett, it's good to see you" Holding his hand out to shake mine warmly, his smile genuine and caring.

"Hi Doc. It's good to see you" I replied.

"How have you been?" He asked.

"Good thanks. I hope you are doing ok?" I replied.

"Yes. Well, listen, I've checked through the images from today and everything looks great. There's no swelling, no new bleeding. You have the scar tissue from the last episode but that's like a scar on your skin, it will always be there. You're a success story!" I could tell he really enjoyed speaking these words.

"Oh great! Thanks Doc." I was deeply relieved to hear that all looked well in the crucially important retina images. He then clicked through images of both eyes on the computer screen to show me that nothing had changed. The images came up on the wall screen just in front of us but I really could not tell if they looked the same or not.

"You can see here (pointing to dark circles) the cell damage from the Cone-Dystrophy, but nothing has changed from last time, and your visual acuity is good" he stated encouragingly.

I thought it a good time to mention my brother's parallel experience.

"One development is that my brother has to undergo retina tests. His doctor told him he had 'holes' in his retinas." I told him to indicate the possible genetic connection to my retina problems.

"I See, that could be a number of things" he said after a brief pause.

"He has to wait until mid-February for his appointment to find out what exactly it is" I added.

"Where is he?"

"London!"

"Oh ok. Well that's a long wait. Keep me posted on what happens with that." He switched the topic deftly back to me. I had no easy way to keep him posted, as I had no direct email to him.

"Have you noticed anything different since last time?"

"Well I have been experiencing a lot of eye fatigue. I am back to full-time teaching and just got done grading 50, 15 page papers" I shared.

"I don't know how you do it!" he responded.

"Well, I enjoy them" I clarified.

"No, no! I don't know how you do it *physically*," he said, orienting me back to the eyes as the topic.

"Well my eyes were really, really tired" I added.

"I bet" he replied and went on to explain that the brain constantly wants the eye to focus when it receives a blurry image. This results in the lens muscles becoming exhausted as they are constantly trying to adjust. He had a name for it and said there was a medication but that it also had side effects relating to glare problems. The eye could not adjust to quick changes in light intensity on the medication. I did not want to live with more side effect dangers. So it looked like eye fatigue would be a constant hazard for me, given the centrality of reading to my job.

He then told me that he felt comfortable, if I did, for me to extend my return to six months instead of three. I told him if he thought I would be ok then we would do that. I trusted his judgment. He gave me a sheet of paper to hand to Claire at the front desk, and we moved to leave the room together. It was a great meeting with good news at its core.

As I left the consulting room, he reiterated that I should check the grid on the web site frequently, which I actually rarely did, and be in touch if anything changed with my vision. He wished me a happy early thanksgiving. I approached Claire's counter and handed her the sheet he had given me to give to her. April seemed like a long time, but I was thrilled that things might be stable enough not to come back for six months. Claire booked me in for April 26th at 9:30 am. I was conscious of the elderly gentleman, wearing both suspenders and a belt on his old Sears jeans, who was coming for another injection right after thanksgiving had stood in this very spot, right in front of Claire, just a few minutes ago. He and his daughter flashed through my mind momentarily as I left with my good news lifting my spirits. I had a good sense of how they might be feeling about being in the midst of their struggles as I breezed home under the cover of heavy cloud. I had been there and, for now at least, I was not anymore.

Sharing the Personal News

That Sunday on the phone I shared the good news with my younger brother, and dad, who were both pleased for me. Dad reiterated that David would have to wait several more months, and we reinforced that we were all concerned that it was such a long wait for him. We swung our collective family worry over from me to him for now.

I took another opportunity to talk to students about my experiences when I did a guest spot in our graduate level communication theory class on the evening of October 29th. To give them something tangible to work with, I shared several conversations from my vision loss journey so far—one I had with Vic and Lisa at the clinic and one with Dad. They were engaged with the topic—looking for potential theory and research questions implied by the conversations. How were these conversations "beautiful?"; what about them was "supportive communication?"; what current theories can explain the connections and sharing of commonalities created within the conversation with Vic a person who, up until that conversation, was a complete stranger?; what theories could explain why my father would offer to give me one of his eyes? We went with the free flowing ideas generated around the table as we unpacked the conversations.

Several also shared from their own lives. One student had a grandfather who had macular degeneration. He had believed his time in the navy during WW2 was causative—especially his time in Japan after the atomic bombs were dropped. Perhaps the exposure was a factor? It was in his story at least. She seemed proud that he had memorized all of the streets in his hometown of Savannah GA such that he maintained relative independence into his later years. Another student shared that she has a relational partner with a different eye disease from mine but that she had similar fears of his complete vision loss. She shared with us how she had thought long and hard about her potentially shifting role to caregiver if the worst were to come true. Questioning the relational partners of vision loss victims for their experiences and responses, I thought, would be a valuable area to explore. Partners' narratives could teach us much about supportive and caring communication. Another said she almost cried when I shared my father's comments about giving me one of his eyes if he could. It was, for me, a beautiful and warm, even intimate, conversation with these bright young scholars.

I was heartened by their response and their ability to connect and relate my experience to their own, and to their current journey into theory and theorizing. I left with a renewed belief that students, perhaps more so graduate students, could learn some valuable lessons about the power and beauty of communication in a traumatic journey centered on the ocular. We would know more as I continued the research and perhaps might even teach a class in communication and disability studies in the spring of 2013. Would anyone sign up who was genuinely interested in the topic, I wondered? Or, would I just get a room full of people needing an upper level class to graduate, or who simply heard that Kellett is a good teacher?! Perhaps, as with any course topic, it would be a diverse mix—a few already curious, and many more to engage, win over, and convince.

Taking Stock: The Difficult, the Odd, and the Awkward

Towards the end of the semester, I began to think about how I had performed my job given where I was with vision loss at this point. My mind began to pinpoint and relive moments where things were difficult or awkward—where I struggled. There were several moments of struggle. Reading the book I used for the classes was sometimes difficult. "Positive Communication" had small and somewhat feint print. I used a magnifying glass sometimes; the moments when reading a paper to give a grade and the paper was out of focus for me—on several occasions I had to wait for my eyes to clunk into focus; the eye fatigue from the huge grading bulges from teaching two writing intensive classes was exhausting.

I was making it through, but I also noticed how much fine detail vision was central to my everyday life of teaching. Teaching was almost as much a non-verbal communication process as it was a verbal one. Responding to a puzzled look with an offer for more clarification; using eye contact to affirm a point with someone; greeting students with eye contact; connecting with students in the everyday way in which they had a relationship with me—each one of them related to me in a slightly different way and the particularities of that unique relationship was very visual; gauging where we were in terms of how well they were understanding and how much I might be boring them with something they already understood—did I need to move on or dwell more on something?; developing a relationship with each of them by face and name; seeing a hand go up for a question and not leaving someone out; spotting those who were drifting off and needed pulling back into the discussion; spotting those who were text messaging or web surfing and asking them to stop; seeing them smile and laugh and sometimes get excited at the discussion; seeing them support each other and occasionally roll their eyes at each other's comments; noticing which of them had personal histories that preceded this class; seeing which students were listening and engaged, and those who appeared not to care; managing the classroom technology which I mostly avoided because of the fine details of the commands and buttons on the equipment; taking attendance, were all more or less everyday activities that were intensively visual in nature. How would I adjust these important functions if things deteriorated more? I knew that I loved seeing them and interacting with them, getting to know them as people, and sensing them and their connection to me, the discussion, and to learning, *visually*. I could not imagine not being able to recognize them and relate to them through sight. How would this work? I knew people did—there were blind professors out there—but it would be a massive relearning process for me, and would necessitate almost quantum shifts in assumptions and behavior for them.

There were visual moments, often seemingly trivial or silly that I enjoyed and that I would miss deeply if I could not have them in the same way anymore.

There were several times when we just laughed as a class at something we said. Seeing the contagious moment of fun capture everyone's expression was a joy. Seeing people connect with ideas and come to life with an example from their lives was a joy …

In early October, Chrissy, from my Positive communication class was talking about changing her hair from blond to auburn just before class started. I participated in the discussion by encouraging her to try it, and that I thought auburn would suit her. They got a kick out of the fact that I shared an opinion. I enjoyed participating in their world just for a moment!

Ari and Lauren dancing in their seats as we connect songs we all knew to the conflict stories we were analyzing. I enjoyed seeing the changing seasons marked by shifts in students' clothing. The boots and sweaters of fall and winter they were obviously looking forward to wearing as soon as they could. Sometimes they came out a little sooner than really needed as if urging the seasons to change.

Fish's hair-cut in November was a major clean up job. He was graduating and interviewing for jobs. I did the same thing when I was about to graduate almost thirty years ago! I joked with him about being a clean cut college kid. The beauty of youth and the bare young skin of August. Sometimes I caught the comments between students about me. For example one day Mara'nta and Morgan were commenting back and forth on something I was wearing—my watch or shirt I think. The moment of recognition as a story being analyzed hits home for someone. Their need for positive feedback and well-timed enthusiasm from me was obvious from visual cues from them. A certain look as if to ask, "Well, did you like my story or anecdote?"

I also had odd moments. The moments when my vision fuzzed out as I was taking attendance for my 11 am Conflict communication class, meaning that I could not read the names momentarily; the moment in my 2 pm positive communication class when Hannah, who was taking two classes with me, looked at me with a puzzled expression as I looked slightly over her face in order to see her face clearly as I spoke to her; the many moments when I walked into chairs and desks that did not register to me as being there, and seeing students chuckle at my clumsiness; the moment when I shared part of my story with my Positive Communication class and to see wide variety of their reactions—VJ texting someone under the desk indifferent to my story, and Damian looking at me as if to ask, "Hey, is this on the test?" and others such as Mallory and Katja look concerned and even shocked by my disclosure.

As the semester came into its final month, I realized I have not been very active on Tate Street, the street adjacent to campus where people met for lunch or coffee. The coffee shops and restaurants carried on fine without me, but I realized I had adjusted my habits into a tight routine of well-worn paths. I brought my lunches which I ate in my office, and worked from home much more. This shift also had to do with not being department head anymore, not needing to be a visible presence around campus anymore, and having less meetings, but I realized I had cut down on everyday activities that required me to navigate menus and crowds.

Daylight savings time came and my mind slipped back to the awful experience of last year when I now believe the macular swelling really accelerated. I remember the sick feeling I had in PF Chang's, and the sense of disorientation I ascribed to the time change at that time. Frustratingly then, I could not explain what was happening to me. I had no such reaction this year. I enjoyed the extra hour in the morning which seemed to last for a whole week. This, to me, confirmed that the real problem with my right eye began about this time last year. A year later now, at the same time, I had adapted quite well. I was not feeling as much dread as I did then for the impending darkness of winter, and the difficulty driving that came with it.

There were moments that reminded me that I could not see well even if in my mind I was feeling like I could. As the mornings grew darker with winter approaching, my Monday, Wednesday, Friday drive to the gym at 6:45 am with Art was essentially in the dark. One morning I sat at the stop sign to turn left onto Lawndale Drive. As usual, I had the windows rolled down to see better. It seemed like a particularly dark and blurry morning though. Perhaps it was the humidity, but headlights were very fuzzy, and it was difficult to judge how far cars were away. I thought I had lots of room to pull out in front of the cars coming from the right. Apparently someone was closer or moving much faster than I could judge and, as I merged into the traffic, someone behind me pressed their horn long enough—for several seconds—to let me know they were very angry at me for pulling out in front of them. My reaction was to question Art about how someone could be so angry, or in such a hurry, at this time of the morning. I was trying to shift the issue onto the other driver, but I do not think Art was convinced. I think he was quietly wondering if he was safe being a passenger in my car! Moments later on the same road Art said, "There's someone in the road!"

I didn't react as I was not sure what he meant and I could not see anyone crossing the street if that was what he meant.

"There's someone stopped *in the road*!" he said more urgently and then, suddenly, I saw a stationary car in my lane with its hazard lights blinking and the driver climbing out. I hit the brakes urgently and passed them safely in the left lane. It was a close call though. It made me realize that I had not seen something important which Art had seen long before I did. I could tell he was concerned. I said something about hoping the other driver was alright and how it sucks to break down when you are trying to get somewhere. Deflect the topic as I did, it did not change the fact that I just could not see very well and these moments, just seconds apart, were a poignant reminder of that fact. "You're not getting better, you've just gotten used to where you are," I reminded myself silently. Mid-way through the workout, at around 7:30 am, I looked outside and was thankful that it was finally daylight.

The period leading up to thanksgiving was relatively calm overall. Classes were going well and, apart from a few odd moments waiting for my eyes to come into focus to share data from a chart, or read something from my notes, and the fatigue of reading and grading, all was well. I was really enjoying teaching again full time and had adjusted to the visual challenges. Our faculty meetings on the other hand were so infrequent that I never really got used to the dynamics of not seeing well in that context, and there seemed to be difficult moments in each of them. One moment in a faculty meeting was difficult but comical in its own way. I was seated at the other end of the table from the department head. During the discussion, we touched on the upcoming self-study process the previous one of which I was in charge. He directed a question my way only with eye contact as the indicator that it was directed at me. There was an uncomfortable gap while I realized he was addressing me with a question. I simply stated that I could not tell he was addressing me, but should I explain that verbal cues to indicate that a question is directed my way would be better than non-verbal which I could not see very well? Should I be educating my colleagues on the limits and assumptions of visually oriented communication? In the fog of the last few weeks of the semester and the busyness of repainting and refinancing the house it slipped as a priority, and I said nothing. Besides, I assumed that they did not particularly care. I knew that, as faculty, we lived largely in our own little bubble worlds.

There was one other awkward moment from that mid-November meeting that made me ponder how I should handle things communicatively. We had begun a tradition a few years before of swapping books with each other at the end of the fall, in lieu of gifts. The date was set for reading day (the day after the end of the semester, and just before exams began). But I did not read small format paperback books any more. I had given all of the ones I still had recently in boxes to the Goodwill, and did not plan on collecting any more.

I did all such reading now on my I-Pad. But what should I do? Explain my non-participation to everyone and cast an unnecessary awkwardness over the event? Buy a used book and participate, knowing that I would never read the book I received? Not show up to the event without any explanation, and risk being gossiped about? I did not know what I wanted to do, and how much I wanted to share. I put off making a decision on this until there might be a reminder come out from someone about the event. It was still a couple of weeks away and there were lots of other things on which to focus my energy. As it turned out I had an excuse for not going. I was on a search committee for Conflict and Peace Studies and that day we were hosting an interview candidate. I was therefore tied up with a dinner appointment. I could have made the book exchange event and the dinner, but I used the interview obligation as a convenient excuse for not participating in the book exchange. I did send an email explaining the need to focus on hosting the candidate, and no one responded. Several others also made excuses for not being there—probably some of them were half-truths too.

As we began discussing the upcoming self-study process as a department, another communication dilemma came up. In his overview of the process, the department head used the word "vision" to capture the experience and process of moving the department forward, as in "… I also believe we can build a strong vision for how to move forward (Nov 12th email) …" Should I request us not to use a term that was, for me, inappropriate? Should I share my preference for us not to use this word to the head and/or to the whole faculty? I had never liked the term given that it privileges one sense over others, and given that it is a borrowed term from the corporate world which in turn borrowed it, clumsily I feel, from religious discourse. I was not convinced any of those layers of borrowing worked well. Corporate leaders may like to think of themselves as receiving visions that help them lead their people into a promised land of success, but this rhetoric stretched beyond thin when applied to a state university setting. We worked essentially in a state bureaucracy where visionary leadership was less realistic than smart progressive goal setting. Not as exciting an image, perhaps, but certainly more realistic. Eight years ago I used the term "destination" as the image of the place we were evolving towards instead of "vision" thinking it much less problematical. In the end, I said nothing about the current use of the term "vision", thinking that I should avoid appearing to lecture the new department head. It would not go over well with him, and others were likely to misinterpret it as me trying to act like I was still in charge of the department. My motto this year was to keep a low profile, avoid politics, and do my own thing. Perhaps there would be a good moment early in the upcoming talks that would be a more natural opportunity to discuss the word and its limitations.

Another poignant moment in a faculty meeting occurred after several colleagues came back from a conference held in Orlando FL.—aka Disneytown! At the end of the meeting one colleague, Loreen, joked that the Disney presence in the place was so all encompassing that she could not even find breath mints that were not in the image of Disney characters! As she shared this, she slid a mint over to me across the table. Several of us in the conversation chuckled. I picked up the mint and tried to see which character it was. I think it was Pluto but I was not sure. It did not really matter. I laughed and let the moment go by without comment, as I did for many similar moments.

I did share the details of my eye condition with a couple of faculty when the need arose, but only when I felt that the need arose. To set up my visit to Roy's graduate communication theory class I met with him over a sandwich and a beer, and talked through the plan that I would be talking to his class about my new project on visual impairment and communication. He was interested in the topic, even talking about possible collaborations. He shared that he had a grandmother who was blind and lived with his family until she died. In addition he had an honors student exploring the experience of deaf holocaust camp survivors. There were some connections, he thought, of sensory loss victims to holocaust survivor narratives that he had been collecting for several years. We might talk later about these connections. I sent him the name of Jacque Lusseyran, a blind holocaust survivor and author, and he sent me the power point presentation of his student studying deaf survivors.

One day (November 1st) I bumped into Jody, a long term colleague, coming out of the department office as I was going in. We had a brief chat—the first of the semester, which was now almost over. I think I surprised her when I told her that I was really enjoying teaching full time again and working from home. She looked shocked when I told her I did not miss the headship role. She told me that she waved to me in the corridor of my building recently but that I had my glasses off and did not respond to her. She joked that I must be "blind" given that I did not see her. I apologized for not responding to her, and asked how she was doing and passed through the awkward conversation-in-the-doorway moment as best as I could, without getting into explanations of my eye conditions. The department office area was not a place to share anything personal. I did follow up with her on email when I got back to my office and explained that I had been in treatment for macular disease and that face recognition problems are a symptom. She responded, sharing from her own life (which I will keep confidential), and then shared the following:

"I don't know about you, but my whole life perspective has changed in the past several years—much of it due to the aging process and how that changes priorities ..."

I responded by agreeing with her, and explaining how my priorities have changed due to my condition:

"Yes I agree. My focus is on what I need to get done and say with the good time/eyesight I have (left). I am happy teaching and doing my own thing as I hope you are ... I am letting so much go around the department ..."

She did not respond further, but I assume she understood and empathized. We had managed to share a rare connection around how health and aging changed our work priorities. It was good to agree on a practical ethos—do not get sucked into the small stuff that is always part of department politics, when you can use the time you have in a much more personally and professionally productive way.

Being Fortunate

That Christmas, I enjoyed putting up the tree again, although it did not feel as special as last year. We also made our trip to the beach, although Hema drove this time. I did not insist on driving to prove that I could. Because I was in a period of stability, the moments were less poignant or heavy to me than last year. I was not thinking that this may be the last time I might be able to decorate and enjoy the tree. I was not thinking that this might be the last winter sunrise I might see coming up over the ocean, and I think we enjoyed these moments more because of the lessening worry. Looking back on last year I wondered should I have been more optimistic and assumed the best scenario, as Hema always urged me to do. Should I have been less dramatic? There were weeks where I did not journal my experience, as I was busy enjoying everyday life and where I was visually. I did not dwell on it as much. But even during this period of stability I knew in the back of my mind all the time that the stability of my vision was a delicate balance, and that things could quickly change for the worse at any time. This existential anxiety was always present for me, but it was pushed into the background in the busy but happy reorganization efforts needed to have Hema move into my house at the end of January. Everybody seemed happy for us as we shared the news of moving in, and our spring wedding plans with close friends and family.

On December 25th I got an email from my brother, David: "Happy Christmas. I hope all is well. Finally got an appointment for my test results on my eyes—end of Feb! Good old NHS speed!"

"Happy Christmas. Yes all's well … Glad the appointment came through. That is slow but you'll know what's happening soon. Hope its best news possible …" I responded.

It was unbearably slow, I know, and I hoped he did not suffer needless vision loss waiting for the National Health Service to grind around to his case, but dwelling on that was pointless. It was Christmas after all, and he had no control over their speed. He had already hustled an early appointment by calling constantly for a cancellation, so he was advocating for himself as much as he could. I knew it would be good for him to at least have a name for his condition, an explanation, and possibly a course of treatment, so I focused on that part of the process. At the same time I could not help but feel fortunate that my condition was caught and treated immediately. I know that many, many souls out there around the world were not so fortunate.

On a slightly lighter note, one day in early February I accidently wore brown socks with black shoes, a black jacket, and a black belt to work. Not the end of the world, I know, and probably not particularly noticeable among the professoriate, but it was unsettling nevertheless. I had an inkling that they were mismatching when I sat down in the office early that morning to prep for upcoming classes. I compared them to my shoes back and forth, and then to my black leather jacket, but I could not quite decide if they were black or dark brown. Assuming they were mismatched, as I knew they were not quite perfectly matched, I hid it as much as possible while in my classes. If I stood upright the whole time they would not see, I told myself. I do not know if anyone noticed, but I remember sitting up on a table as a student talked and then jumping down because I could see that my socks were visible. It was odd not to be able to tell definitively what color the socks were, but I knew that my students would see the difference if they were looking. I had not noticed color blindness up until this point and, perhaps, I was seeing the signs of this creeping in, as all the literature I read on Cone-Dystrophy had predicted.

Even in early February, as the first daffodils popped up in the front yard, and thoughts turned to Valentine's Day gift shopping, I began noticing the slight brightening of the morning and evenings. The days were getting a little longer, and there would be less of a struggle for me with driving in the dark. The talk between Hema and me began to focus on plans to get married in May, and on hoping that many family members from England and India would make it for the events. Classes were going well. Hema had moved in and we were enjoying life together in the same space. It was not without its tensions and adjustments but, overall, things were morphing together well. The house was beginning to reflect a melding of both of our styles. Western Mid-century modern meets South India. Our house was becoming a sort of metrosexual—pooja space, bachelor black leather meets earthy lotus carving; Ganesh meets Natuzzi; curls of exotic incense wafting around the west elm shelving; Delicious curry served in Williams-Sonoma dishes. Somehow it worked visually and aesthetically, as it did for us relationally. People enjoyed coming to our home. We complemented each other well. We enjoyed having people over for amazing Indian food, or just watching back to back episodes of The Mentalist, and Castle together by ourselves.

A large pile of boxes full of things that she just could not find room for in the house sat stacked several high in the sun room—leaving just enough room for a walkway through. It had me joking several times about calling the television show "Hoarders" so they might feature us in an episode, commentary that Hema did not find amusing or sensitive. She had worked tirelessly to get her things packed up and moved to our house. But there just was not room anywhere for the contents of these very last two carloads that we brought home on that strange tornado threatening stormy winter night, just before her lease ran out on the last day of January. Yet, one of the key differences between us was now starkly visual—she kept almost everything—not finding the time to get rid of things, and I kept almost nothing—not finding the time to hold onto things. She had a story attached to almost every paper and object in her many boxes. I had forgotten most of what I used to own—preferring the lightness of space and clean lines to what I thought was clutter, and the heaviness of unnecessary memory. But on that difference, I would have to be understanding. We struggled to meet in the middle. She was moving into what was my single person space, and that is rarely easy. She did not need me criticizing what she thought of as meaningful things she was bringing with her. She agreed to have a major clear out of unnecessary things as long as I could be patient and not make comments that made her feel pressured on the issue. Progress would be made if I could wait until there was a good block of time to tackle this major task. It was a deal.

After a faculty meeting in which I had my I-Pad with me in its bright pink cover, one colleague commented that my cover looked, "metro-(sexual)" chuckling as he made the comment. I guess pinkish red was a little surprising to him for an I-Pad cover. I laughed with him. Why not, I thought? In truth, I chose red because my furniture was black leather and devices with black covers disappeared into the furniture. I lost my phone this way quite frequently. The only two choices in the store were black and red.

The morning after Valentine's Day, I went to the gym and worked out alone. Art and Jon were otherwise engaged. For the first time Chris and I chatted alone for a few minutes. He had just had an injection and we discussed the fact that he was now having injections in both eyes, alternating every two weeks. I felt for him. He needed cataract surgery but they could not do that until this treatment was over, and there was no specific end point for this treatment. They had no idea how long it would take to stabilize the decline. He was in a tough scenario, yet we chatted about how fortunate we were to have some treatment available, and that it was making a difference. He told me about his cousin who has the same problem. He was a school bus driver and when the lines on the road became wavy, he knew his time in that job was done. He turned in his keys and retired. The well-ordered world of straight lines that a bus driver relies on was changing forever for him. Chris acted out the scene of passing his keys to some imaginary supervisor. We both understood the frightening and unsettling experience of seeing the wavy road lines. It was a sad moment in his cousin's life, given that it essentially ended his career. Sadder still must have been the moment when the doctor told him they could not give him an injection. Chris did not know why. Perhaps his eyes were too far gone to rescue. Perhaps there was some other issue which meant that injections would have been more dangerous than helpful. Neither of us knew the actual story. But, for a moment, we imagined the devastation of being told his condition was essentially untreatable, and we immediately felt fortunate ourselves. We both said so, lingering on the words and repeating them several times—knowing that we could have been telling a very different story, one just like his cousin. His cousin could now see very little, and was disabled. That could have been us very easily by now, and we both knew it. Chris ended the conversation by saying that never in a million years did he ever imagine being in the situation of fighting for his sight. I mirrored the same sentiment. I had thought it so many times. We laughed briefly and then we were back to working out, acutely aware of the curious mix of bad luck and good luck that we both lived with, as we briefly shared our common storylines of being fortunate—*this is not what we imagined … but it could be much worse.*

That spring semester I enjoyed what I felt was a period of relative stability. It seemed like a long time until Friday April 26th when I would have to go back for my six month check-up. Being busy with wedding plans (May

25th), and enjoying another good semester of teaching and writing, and with hopefully no more injections looming, I put the fear and trepidation mostly to the back of my mind. I focused on enjoying myself and developing my writing on the topic of vision loss and communication. That spring, I wrote the first academic paper focusing on my experiences of vision loss. The paper entitled, "Mutually supportive communication and relational narratives: Online conversations between two friends in declining health" documents the conversations between myself and my friend Bud Goodall who was dying of cancer, and the powerful impact of those conversations in helping me cope with the process. I sent the paper to the National Communication Association Conference with a hope that it might be accepted to be presented in DC in November. I mention this because it was my first real public account of my experience. I also sent the paper to several colleagues who I thought would be interested but, oddly, I heard back from no one. Perhaps they were too busy. I followed that paper quickly with an essay entitled, "Toward a framework for the study of communication and ocular health and disease: A personal narrative of vision loss." The essay, for a book chapter on health communication, would tell some of my own story so far, and use my story to develop a research agenda centered on ocular health and disease. I was exhausted at the end of the year, but committed myself to writing the essay.

I also became much more open and proactive in talking with my classes about being visually impaired. I even joked several times about it when accidentally crashing into a table that I did not quite see, or if I had a hard time reading my notes in front of them. Several responded with curious questions. I remember Christina asking me after class one day what exactly was wrong with my eyes, and after I told her the names of the conditions, she followed up with the question, "So is there a chance that you might lose your sight, like, *be blind?*"

"Yes there's a chance," I replied, not knowing how to articulate the chances to her in any specific way. The question hung heavy as we stood in the classroom momentarily alone, and then we were quickly off to our respective tasks—she to her next class and me to my office hour. I appreciated her curiosity and caring interest.

One particularly touching moment occurred in my CST 207 (Relational Communication) class. One evening I talked briefly about the impact of my impairment on relationships to others, and on my ability to read print and handwriting and non-verbal communication. Shortly after this I was grading their relational journals. There was a note attached to the front of the journal of Cailey, a smart, sensitive, and caring Sign-language major. She wrote: "Dr.

Kellett, I rewrote most of my journal in clearer handwriting because I know you have had problems with your eyes. I hope this helps." I was so touched by this. She had rewritten by hand probably 30 pages of journal notes and entries so that I could read it more easily. Undoubtedly her connection to disability studies had given her a deepened sense of empathy to me, and it really showed. It made me realize that teaching is so much about developing caring relationships, and sometimes the care is expressed mutually to great effect.

One afternoon in my office I shared a joke with my graduate advisee Tessa. I had given her a copy of the paper I wrote detailing the impact of supportive communication on my journey into visual impairment, so she knew a good bit about my condition. I was explaining to her how sometimes faces appear blank to me, and that I sometimes cannot see people who are waving to me from a distance. It is very easy for those people to misunderstand as rudeness or indifference. As if on cue, someone walked by my office door and paused and waved momentarily. I knew it was a female, most likely one of my students, but beyond that I did not have a clue as to who she was. I waved back and said, "Hi there." As the person walked away, I told Tessa that I had no idea who it was. We shared the inside joke, and laughed together.

The first half of the semester taught me a valuable lesson, which I listened to. Reading the huge number of pages necessary to teach and grade papers from my students often left me with painful eye fatigue. I had to rest them frequently, and also had to orchestrate lighting and context carefully to read papers. Going into the last round of grading for the semester which would involve 50 × 15 page papers, 20 × 5 page papers and 20 × 15 page journals I decided it was time to go paperless. With the help of Hema, we set up e-drop boxes so that I could read everything on my well-lit computer screen where I could enlarge the pages I would have to read. It was time to be proactive in maximizing the technology I had available to me, and it felt like a positive move not only in saving paper, but in saving my eyes!

· 11 ·

SIX MONTH CHECK-UP

April 26th 2013

During the week of my follow up exam, I began to visualize sitting in the waiting room and going through the battery of tests all over again. I thought about the banal water feature for the first time in months. I remembered the sights, sounds, and smell of the doctor's office. How it was organized, and how people moved through its spaces and rooms. I pictured the Christmas tree that I have seen there a couple of times now. I wondered who would still be working there. I was both mildly nervous, and fairly confident at the same time. The appointment would mark approximately two years since my first diagnosis and the beginning of this journey. I was hopeful. I figured I was lucky to be able to still do what I could do. I was thankful. I was getting inspired to write more about the experience so far. I was happy. I checked the weather and became a little anxious that it would be such a bright sunny day. Gray would have been perfect for driving home, but I had done it before and I knew I would be fine.

The Appointment and Cautious Optimism

The evening before my appointment I decided what I would order for Hema's wedding ring. It matched her engagement ring of light blue sapphire and diamonds in white gold. Momentarily, I remembered back to the time I bought her engagement ring. I was wondering and worrying about the unanswerable questions of how long I would be able to see it clearly, and for how long would I be able to see her clearly? I still could see both quite well. I might have to look slightly over the top, or just to the side, to focus on the details of the ring, or her face, but we had come to accept this as an integral part of everyday life. It was a far, far, better reality than what might so easily have been by this point.

The morning of the appointment I worked out and then met Hema at home by 8:15 am before she went to work. She told me I looked nervous, that it was "written all over my face." I could not argue with her. Truthfully, I was nervous. They might find something new, requiring a second course of injections. There might be signs of trouble ahead that I could not sense on an everyday level. The uncertainties were heavy in this moment. She gave me a quick pep talk: "You don't need to worry. I know I don't completely understand. I know I can't, but you need to stop worrying. You're going to be fine … as long as I am here you're going to be fine."

Her encouragement helped, even though I could not remember all that she said that morning. I was nervous about the brightness of the morning, and tuned a lot of the talk out. The day was cloudless and bright, too bright to drive home dilated, but I took both my clip-ons and my Smith Optics sunglasses. Before I left the house, I put them both on and looked at myself in the mirror. I looked odd, really odd—glasses on top of glasses, but I wanted to be prepared to make it home without struggling with the light. Perhaps I should just get a welders mask I thought, playfully.

While checking in at the front desk which was staffed by two new people, Clare turned around from a computer at the back of the reception area and said "hi." I said "hi" back, and I was glad that she remembered me. Almost immediately after sitting down and looking around at my fellow patients, then at the bland landscape pictures on the walls, my name was called. It looked remarkably quiet today, and it was good to get moving through the stages quickly. First was the obligatory letter test, which I always dreaded. My right eye struggled until I found a place to look just above the letters from where it was easier to read them. My left eye washed out completely at first and saw nothing, but then it gradually came into focus and I could follow down to about where I could six months ago. My mind slipped away to the possibility of taking this test at the DMV. I noted to myself that they were very unlikely to give my eyes time to "warm up" and come into focus, as they did here at the retina clinic. I felt that I had to adapt and strategize more to see the letters clearly than last time. I ended up about at the same place as last time, but it was more work, and slower going. I focused on staying relaxed so that my blood pressure would not go up and possibly limit my vision. I asked for feedback, and the new technician told me that they were about the same as last time. Then came the stinging dilation drops, and I was quickly off to wait for the retina photographs. Again things moved quickly and I was through that and waiting for Dr. Sanders in an examining room within a few minutes. There were some new pictures on the monitors. Lush forests with well-worn paths through them were interspersed with the usual microscopic nature images. They were all beautiful, vibrant images that seemed to revel in and even celebrated the visual—the amazing world of nature through the eyes. I also noticed a new "Wet AMD at a Glance" poster in the room on the wall to my left. It had images comparing normal and diseased retinas, along with pictures of a child's face as if seen through "normal" eyes, and those of someone with advanced macular degeneration. I could see both well, so I was comforted to know that I was doing fine, but the advanced images were scary. Large sections of the persons face were pearly white foggy blankness.

Dr. Sanders came in with a big hello and a hand shake. He was quick to tell me that he was very pleased with the results of the six month follow-up. He told me that things appeared stable and that, unless something changed significantly, he would see me again in one year. He asked me what questions I had, as if to move the meeting towards ending. If I did not have any questions then we were done. I was a success story and they were happy to let me go now. We chatted briefly again about my research ideas relating to vision loss. I told him that I had begun writing papers about the experience, and that I would still like to follow up with him on using his patient contacts. He told me to let him know what I needed. I also told him about my brother's test results and, after cringing a little at how slow his treatment seemed in the UK, he told me he would love to examine him if he is ever here visiting. Twins are fascinating specimens to ophthalmologists given the genetic connection to etiology. Without more questions for him I was quickly on my way. Before I left the nurse told me: "We're here if you need us."

It was a sweet and caring thing to say. I told her it was good to see her again, and I could tell she liked to be remembered too. She was the nurse who first took my retina images two years ago and, to help me relax a bit, told me I looked like Pauly Shore. It was a poignant au revoir given everything that had happened between those two moments. Would the third year ahead bring more stability as this second one had? Would the story take an unexpected and dramatic change of direction as it did early in the first year? Would the swelling problem return? They could, very easily. What lessons about communication and relationships would the year ahead teach me? I was curious and open to it. Within a few seconds of being told that they would give me a call close to a year from now, I was on my way—out into the blazing light of the late morning in spring-time to engage the year head-on and find out.

A Reality Check

As if by way of a reality check from all of the good news, on the very next Monday morning—a rainy dingy morning—I was driving alone to the gym at 6:45 am and saw a person on a bicycle peddling in the rain just in time to swerve around them. They were wearing dark clothes and nothing reflective, and yet they were peddling stoically in the middle of the lane. It was a wake-up call literally, and metaphorically, that morning. My eyes were now wide open at this early hour. My immediate reaction was to think how stupid of them to be so difficult to see. At least they should wear a reflective vest, or have a reflector on the back of the bike, I thought. They had nothing to indicate they were on the road. Then I thought, how quickly life would change if I hit someone in this way—reflective vest or not. This would be a minor detail if I actually hurt someone. For a dark, selfish, moment I imagined some attorney investigating me and finding out that I should not be driving at all after critically injuring his client. The finale to his case was to craftily expose me in court as someone who is driving with knowledge that they should not be behind the wheel of a car. Each question gradually leads me into a corner where I cannot escape the guilt.

The incident almost happened right by my optometrists office on Lawndale Avenue. I reminded myself that she had told me I was still legal to drive, and even felt confident that she was sharing the road with me, so I shook off the imaginary but scary court room drama scene and pressed on to the gym. Again, just for a moment, I imagined having to take a cab or get a ride everywhere and it was, as ever, a miserable thought. Just a little longer, just a little longer, please Lord, just a little longer. These were the near misses, the worries, the rationalizations, and the hopes of a liminal driver, and I knew it.

There were still a few weeks left before the end of the second year of this experience, and they would be filled with many hours of reading and screen time. My grading mountain was looming large and so was the research and writing time necessary to complete the two papers I had committed to write before the end of May.

Immediately before graduation, one of my students from last spring, Elena, came by my office to say bye, and to introduce me to her boyfriend. She was a positive person and full of the energy and zest for life. As she stood in my doorway I did not know who she was. I could tell she was hesitant to come in, assuming I did not know her or that I had forgotten her, which would assume she was not important enough to me to remember! All of these layers were immediately present in that moment of hesitation. We quickly moved through it as she walked towards me, but she did check for clarity as she walked in: "Hi Dr. Kellett. Did you not know it was me..?"

YEAR 3

Mid-May 2013 to Early July 2014

· 12 ·

THE SUMMER OF LOVE

In mid-May, Hema's mother and father arrived from India to stay with us. They were coming for our wedding, and to stay with us for about seven weeks in total. I must admit it was a daunting thought to have them in our small house with us, but I was told that Indians rarely come for such a *short* period of time! All things being relative, it was a good opportunity for them to get away from the hustle and bustle of Bangalore, and to see how we lived here in the U.S. It was also an opportunity for Hema to spend real time with them and enjoy their company, and for me to get to know them more closely as my soon to be in-laws.

Night Sight

News of their visit had quickly filtered out into our community of friends, which meant that we had numerous invitations for evenings and dinners with our friends. It also meant a lot of driving at night for Hema, but she thoroughly enjoyed the social gatherings. There were times when I felt bad that she would have to drive so much. Back and forth she drove them to Winston, around Greensboro, to Raleigh, Charlotte, Asheville, Washington DC, and around town in between longer trips. She never complained, although I did fill up her gas tank when she needed it while on one of these trips, and once I asked her to drive them in my car to Winston as hers was really getting used a lot.

One night on our way back from Lata and Nand's house in Winston, Hema was pulling off a road onto an exit ramp to get onto I-40 t to take us back to Greensboro. For some reason my eyes convinced my brain that we were about to hit another car directly from behind, "STOOOOPPPP!" I shouted, filled with the almost paralyzing terror of an impending impact that might have been disastrous. I cannot remember being so afraid before. I was pinned back to my seat and breathless with fear. Hema slowed right down and said something along the lines of "what's wrong love, there's nothing in front of us." I had seen the reflection of her headlights bouncing off the reflectors on the corner of the exit ramp fence, and my brain had been convinced by these images that it was another car stopped right in front of us. Literally I was afraid of our own reflection! Perhaps I was also a little afraid of anything going wrong before the wedding, and especially while all four of us were in the car. I was embarrassed to make the mistake in front of my in-laws to be. After a minute or two, I simply said that I could not see well in the dark, and left it at that. They did not say anything, but I did wonder what they must have been thinking—their daughter driving us around, which would be unusual in India, and me seeing things that were not there. They were already experiencing some culture shock in the early part of their visit, and now this strange scene!

On another occasion we were driving home at night and passing a dark field on the passenger side to my right, my eyes convinced me that I was seeing dinosaurs leaping around in the field. I did not say anything this time but I did note to myself that we had, just a day or two earlier, tried to convince her mom and dad to go with us to see the movie, Jurassic Park in 3D. They were not interested in seeing the movie, insisting that they already saw it years before, so we only talked about it briefly. Yet, somehow my eyes were picking up small cues and, when mingled with my own fears and suggestions coming from somewhere in my mind or a recent conversation, again I was seeing things that were not there. These moments made me realize that vision involves both the problem of not seeing things that were there, which is what we might normally expect, and the more curious and strange experience of seeing things that were not there.

On a few other occasions, when I drove us all in the evening, Hema was good about giving me verbal cues to help me supplement what I could not see. Her parents said nothing to me about these practices of coaching me in driving, even though they must have appeared odd to them. One evening I had driven us the short distance to dinner at her friend Agnes's home. She had wanted to cook Hema's parents a traditional meal from her native Hungary—chicken paprikash, and they were happy for the opportunity to try something new, even though they probably would have preferred something spicier. Driving us home I made a series of mistakes. First, I lost track of how to get out of her neighborhood, and thought we were back on the main road when we were still a turn away. When we got on the main road (Elm Street) Hema had to tell me to change lanes to avoid a cyclist who was in the right hand lane—riding at night with no lights. I knew someone was there and I would not have hit him, but she saw him a long time before I did. She was able to get me into the left lane well before we were upon him. When we were driving along Pisgah Church Road I had a hard time seeing that the dark road curved to the right after a long straight stretch, and had to adjust slightly before she noticed. Finally, when the left turn to our neighborhood appeared, she coached me to turn. I was struggling a little to see it in the gloomy light. It is a turn off that is often hard to see in daylight, but at night it is unlit, across three lanes of road, and hidden somewhat by foliage. Of course, to someone with good eyesight, it is easy to see day or night, but for me it was just hard to see it. She told me to always look for the crossing sign as the turn is directly after that. In the course of a mile or so I had several difficult moments. As we made a couple of turns in the neighborhood to get to our house I simply said, "My night vision is getting worse."

"What do you mean," Hema asked?

"I can't see as well at night!" I replied, matter-of-factly. I did not know what else to say, and did not want to get deeper into the topic with her parents sitting in the back seat.

After an enjoyable night at Aggie's, I kept my fears to myself beyond simply stating what I was thinking, but her parents must have been wondering just how bad my eyes were, given the number of problems I had in such a short distance, and Hema's active coaching while I drove. I hoped to myself that they were not wondering what their daughter was getting herself into. I let the moment go without any further discussion, as did Hema. Nobody else raised any questions beyond this fragmentary conversation either. But I knew it was not a good feeling, swirling around in the back of my head, to imagine that soon I might not be able to drive at night at all. I suppressed the thought, and its feelings, and tried to focus on the main task I had for me and Hema's dad—to get the yard in as good a shape as we could before the wedding, and before the weather turned hot. I had bought Hema's dad, "Mr. P" as I called him, a pair of gardening gloves like mine, and he was beginning to wear them to help me prune fig trees, weed the vegetable garden, and mow the yard. It was nice to have some help, he was glad of some activities besides social gatherings, and Indian channel television, to break up the long days, and it was a good bonding time for us guys. Because of his help around the yard I promoted him to "Captain P" and the name stuck ever since.

Over the course of their weeks with us we got into a routine that included all of us watching two of their Indian serials (called prime time soap operas in the US). The shows were melodramatic accounts of Indian family life, which provided me with fascinating insights into their culture as they commented on, and helped me make sense of, the stories and their meanings. We watched two of these shows together almost religiously. They really enjoyed the fact that I embraced their culture, and sat down to watch these shows with them. I did, however, have to sit up close to the screen to see the English subtitles. Hema sat up close with me and her parents must have enjoyed watching us in front of them as a happy couple—watching their shows with them. One day while Hema was out of town, her mother asked me to sit on the couch and watch it with her and her husband. We would all sit together and enjoy the dramas. But I could not see the subtitles from that distance. I quietly explained that I needed to sit up close to the screen so that I could read the subtitles. Nothing more was said about this and they simply accepted that I needed to be up as close as two feet from the screen. The same was true when we watched tennis from Wimbledon together. I had turned the arm chair around and positioned it about two feet from the screen where I could see the details well—like the ball going back and forth. It was just how things were, and they did not say any more about it to me.

Our Wedding and Aftermath

On May 25th the wedding went wonderfully well. I had little or no idea what was coming in the Hindu ceremony but I followed the lead of the priest, and the crowd seemed to enjoy the exotic spectacle. I followed him in reciting words I did not understand. I followed him in placing flowers systematically around a god I did not know. I followed him as he put jaggery (raw sugar) and fennel seeds in my hair, poured milk all over my hands, and had the crowd throw flower petals and rice over us for good luck. It was a delightful balance of earthiness and the spiritual.

Towards the end of the ceremony the priest led us out into the parking lot beside the temple. We were to engage in a brief ritual involving a star that was somehow linked to the auspiciousness of our union. The star was well hidden behind the blazing noon sunlight—I did not quite catch which star and what exactly it meant, but I was supposed to point up to the star as if it were night time, and I was showing it to my wife. It was a bright day and the task of looking up and pointing was unbearable for me. My sunglasses were somewhere in my bag, which was somewhere out of reach at that moment. When called upon, I pointed up somewhere close to where the star might be, but kept my head down. The resulting picture was a comical failure, and not one I enjoyed looking at.

The image made Hema's mother laugh when she was looking through the pictures and videos later. Hema also found it hilarious. It was a week after the wedding and Deepak was over for dinner when we looked through the pictures again. It seemed too soon to be going through them all again but that was on the agenda for the evening, so I had no choice. When we got to the picture of me pointing unconvincingly up to the sky, while bowing painfully away from the sun, Hema's mother laughed loudly. She found the picture comical. Hema laughed with her. I am sure it was quite ridiculous given that she likely had a clear sense of how the moment was supposed to look, and this was far from it. Privately I was a little hurt and offended that neither she nor Hema acknowledged the fact that I had acute sensitivity to bright light. I also knew that they were laughing with me, not at me, in any kind of mean way. They enjoyed making fun of the picture and I held back from saying much. I recognized that it was a comic image, and I could understand them laughing at it. I think Deepak sensed my hurt feelings while they were laughing. We all moved on to have a great evening with Deepak, but the laughter at the picture irritated me.

The same thing happened a week later when we relived all of the pictures again with Pat (our JP), Michael (her husband), and Joyce (a mutual friend and former colleague, now retired). There were a few pictures I would have eliminated from the slide show, but I had very little say in that issue. A week or two later the topic of laughing at the picture came up in conversation. I remember explaining to Hema that I could not look up because of the bright sunlight. Hema gently explained to me that I should not take things so seriously, and that I ought to be able to laugh at the picture. She was right, although part of me was still annoyed at being laughed at in a vulnerable moment. Why was I being overly sensitive, I wondered to myself? How much sensitivity and accommodation is it realistic to expect from a partner of family member (in this case a mother in law who has minimal understanding of my eye problems) in these types of moments and situations? I told myself that it is better to let the moment go, and to simply laugh along. To explain would have made her feel uncomfortable and awkward, and it would have taken the fun out of the moment for her. It might also have helped to organize things around the negativity of my eye problems unnecessarily, and that would have been selfish on my part. The family time during the seven weeks from mid-May to early July had enough turbulent moments without me adding another issue into the mix.

Reshaping my Academic Identity

Amidst the festivities, I kept pushing forward with writing goals. In May I completed my first paper on ocular health and disease that would later be published as a chapter in an edited book on health communication. The chapter outlines an agenda for research which positions ocular health and disease as an important, and neglected, part of health communication. The chapter raised many questions that link eye health to communication. The questions listed in the paper were drawn out of the personal story of my experience of the first year of vision loss. It felt awkwardly personal, but I also needed to make the beginnings of this topic as a course of writing for me. I wanted so much for my story to have a meaning beyond itself, and beyond myself. After completing the paper, I wished I could have told more of the story but I ran out of space and, so, limited it to the dramatic early stages of the first year. Vision loss would become as central a part of my professional identity through this work, as it did my personal life. The reviewer liked the chapter, but was puzzled over whose personal narrative it was that was included as part of the chapter. It was *my* story and I thought I made that clear in the draft. In response to their comments, I made sure there was no doubt about this in the revised version. I was pleased with the paper, and with the moment of career change it represented for me. I was at a point in my career where I wanted only to focus on papers I really wanted to write. I wanted to make a contribution based on *my own experience*—and essentially to turn my loss into something positive. This first little book chapter was an important first step for me.

In mid-June, I left Hema with her parents for a few days, to present a conference paper at the George Gerbner Conference on media and violence in Budapest, Hungary. The paper went well, but I found myself overtaken with fear much of the time, trying to find my way around. I had always been a fairly relaxed and confident traveler, but here I struggled to read the street signs, menus, and see the denominations on the Hungarian currency, which was also foreign to me. I was feeling vulnerable in a place where very few people spoke English enough to help me. I knew I could not even pronounce the street names, which were all only in Hungarian, if I needed help getting back to the hotel.

One morning I walked up to the nearby Arkad (Mall) to look around and purchase some snacks for the room. I tried to remember landmarks that would be useful to finding my way back. The enormous Ikea store on the left, and the even bigger bowling and beer facility just past it, would be on my right coming back. The railway on my right would be on my left. This helped, of course, but I felt strangely anxious. I wandered round the mall not finding much in the way of fruits or snacks for the room. When I did find a small grocery store, they would not take Euro's, and looked shocked when I pulled out a debit card. A sharp "NO GOOD" was all I got in English and I left embarrassed as everyone stared at me. I did find a health food store where they would take a credit card, even though the friendly staff had never swiped one before. Thankfully it worked, and I think they were as surprised as I was that it went through. I stocked up on healthy juices and snacks, so I would not have to wander out much beyond the conference activities. As I exited the mall, I found myself confused and on the verge of panic. Which way was it to go back to the hotel? Momentarily I was lost. Trying not to get too anxious, I crossed the street via the underpass, walked around the other part of the mall area where the outdoor vendors were sitting, selling vegetables by the train ticket kiosk, and eventually found my bearings to the street where my hotel was located. Besides the Ikea and the bowling alley, the rest of the terrain was block after block of banal soviet era apartments, which gave no clues to where you might be if a stranger here. With relief, I found my way back to the correct street. I came to a pedestrian crossing light, which all pedestrians there seemed to obey dutifully, but it had no sounds associated with stopping or crossing as they had evolved to do in the US. It turned green to go, and red to stop, and that was it. As I headed back to the hotel, I could not help but think that this would be a really tough place to be blind.

Jan, a warm and friendly professor from Belgium who I met at the start of the conference, had braved the impressively extensive public transport system the day before, and found his way to downtown to look around and take some pictures of the flooded river. But he said it was not easy. Everything was in Hungarian, and very few people spoke much English outside of the tourist friendly city center. I knew as he told me his story that I would not be so brave, but I did not explain this to him. Another new conference friend, Karin, asked me several times if I had been downtown yet to explore the old touristy part of the city. I simply told her I would look around at the end of the conference, and felt too self-conscious to explain my anxiety over not seeing well enough to jump on a bus or train and guess where to get off. They did not think twice about doing this, but I knew in these moments that their comfortable normality was not mine anymore.

While I was there, and especially when it came to the tourist side of the conference visit, I kept thinking how much more fun it would be if Hema was with me. Actually I was glad much of the time that she was not there. It was a lousy hotel. It was hot weather and the AC did not work. The second floor smelled of old frying oil that drifted up from the kitchen. Worst of all, I came home with my hands covered in lesions from bed bug bites. She would have moved us to a different hotel within about ten minutes of checking into this one! But I know she would have pushed us to get out into the city more to explore. She would not let fear or language barriers and cultural differences hold her back. I was struck by how much I had come to rely on her, her confidence, and energy for life.

The Kindness of Strangers

On the way back home from Budapest I transferred planes in Frankfurt. As I waited a little nervously to board, I decided to rush into the restroom and wash my face and brush and floss my teeth. This was a typical pre-flying anxiety ritual for me, more than any need to clean up per se. I was just standing around and nervously checking and double checking my boarding pass and passport prior to boarding, so this would give me a task to complete to kill a few minutes. I found a bathroom close by and took my glasses off to splash my face and dry it. I placed them on the cramped counter near the sink. I brushed and flossed and pushed my toiletries back into my bag. I felt my own anxiety as I shoved things around in my bad to accommodate my toiletries, and cursed under my breath as they did not seem to fit as well as they had before I took them out. More haste-less speed, as my mother would rightly say! I had no idea why I was so nervous. I think I was just anxious to get home to my new family. In my anxiety and haste to get back into the boarding area, I walked out without my glasses. Intent on boarding, I did not notice that I did not have them on. As I turned the corner to exit the restroom area, I heard a loud voice calling out to me, "Hey, *HEY*, you left your glasses!"

Luckily I realized the statement was calling *me* back. I rushed back in to see them next to the sink where I had left them. The man repeated his statement at a normal speaking volume to indicate that he was the one who had called me back.

"Oh thank you, *thank you so much*. Wow! I need those!" I responded looking directly at the kind stranger and trying to half joke away the relief. He nodded and I quickly put them on and left, saying thank you again as I walked out. As I waited to board the plane my mind flashed through just how much of a mistake it would have been for me to leave them behind, and just how easy it would have been to do that given that we were now boarding. This kind stranger could also quite easily have ignored my mistake and gone on with his travels, never to see me again. But he did not. Even if I had missed my glasses while I was boarding and still able to look for them, there would be no guarantee that in the ensuing panic I would realize I had left them in the bathroom. Momentarily I envisioned the rest of the flight, and the journey home from the airport with Hema, without my glasses. Within an hour I would have had terrible headaches, and would not be able to see much of anything while on the plane. The relief washed all over me as I breathed out a long calm breath and recognized the beauty of the kind choice he made to call me back. He chose to help me. I looked around for the person who had called me back as if I wanted to thank him again but, of course, he was gone. The moment was a quick interconnection of fellow travelers in the fluid impersonality of a foreign airport, but the lesson stayed with me—the less one is able to rely on oneself and ones abilities, the more one will have to rely on the kindness of strangers, and strangers are often kinder than one might expect. Perhaps this would have been good for me to test more while I was in Budapest, where I timidly avoided things that I feared.

Natural Rhythms

The quarter year period leading up to the summer solstice and the longest day of the year had fast become my favorite time of year. The days were longer and lighter, which made driving much easier for me. The solstice always brought mixed feelings for me. It was a long and light time of year, but it heralded the next quarter, and the inevitable shortening of the days that would follow late in the summer quarter and into the fall and winter. These rhythms had taken on a deeper meaning for me, and I felt them now keenly ingrained into my own rhythms of light and dark. On the day of the solstice I had a conversation with friend, JG. I remarked that it felt good to be at the lightest time of year. He responded by saying that this day began "The downward spiral" towards the darkness of fall and winter. It struck me as a particularly negative take on the brightest day of the year. "No, No, No" I said, "lets enjoy the longer days. It will be a while before we notice things getting darker." He agreed, but the moment did make me think of the dark mornings ahead driving to the gym, and the dark evenings ahead driving home from night class. We laughed, but we also knew there was an inevitable cycle to the comings and goings of light and dark. There would be bright and long days for a while to come and they were to be enjoyed.

The "super moon" a couple of days later on June 23rd was really spectacular in the cloudless 10 pm sky. After we had dinner at Lata and Nand's in Winston with a fun group of people, we stepped out into the beautiful early summer evening to drive back to Greensboro in John's car. I was driving back with him and his daughter Milana partly just to get a brief break from the family who all went with Hema, and partly to keep John company on the drive back which was unfamiliar to him. We left the house just before everyone else. The three of us stopped momentarily in the driveway and gazed up at the big bright moon—oohing and ahhing for a minute before the hour long drive back to Greensboro. John asked Milana and me if we could make out the features of the face in the moon. She could, and took joy in pointing them out, and narrating what each feature looked like. I told him that I could not see any of the features, but that I could see that it was bright and beautiful. I always loved the moon, and it was still a wonder to look at. As if processing the words, he thoughtfully repeated what I had just said, that I could not make out any of the facial features. I think it shocked him that, to me, it was essentially a big blank disk in the sky—it was beautiful definitely, but faceless for me. In that moment we shared a common sense of wonder at the beauty of the moon. Yet, the simple vivid difference between us was that for them the moon had a face and for me it did not—at least not one that I could see while looking directly at it.

Newlyweds

On July 3rd we dropped Hema's mother and father off in Raleigh to begin their long journey home to Bengaluru. Earlier that day we were sitting around talking about something related to my eyes. Her mother looked at me earnestly and, in her now much improved English, said maternally: "Eat lots of carrots Pete, and greens. All good for eyes!"

"Thanks Mummy-Ji, I will." I replied, aware and grateful for the genuine care behind this statement, and for the fact that this was one so called "old wives tale" that had a lot of truth to it.

After they left, we were suddenly newlyweds with each other, and had our own house back, all to ourselves. We enjoyed everyday life together enormously—walking, making meals, laughing, being silly, arguing and occasionally being cranky, picking lots of figs, and vegetables from the garden. It was a wonderful bit of summer together after all of the hoopla and family time was over, and before we heard the familiar refrain of "back to school" begin to permeate our realities starting with television advertisements in July.

One day we revisited the idea of making plans to take a short vacation together—a honeymoon of sorts—before school started up again. As usual Hema was full of ideas and was open to mine, which were admittedly much fewer. Early in the discussion I told her that I would prefer somewhere where it would not be a tropical destination with lots of blazing sunshine. Battling that kind of environment would be miserable for me. We agreed upon a short cruise out of New York City around Canada as far as Halifax, Nova Scotia, and back to New York. She wanted to spend a day in NYC which she had never been to so we built that into the plans, although I would rather have taken the earlier flight back after the cruise. As she spent 45 minutes on the phone with the cruise agent making all of the decisions, I sat close by to give my input when needed. But she really did all of the work, as usual. She had asked me to plan something for once when we discussed a honeymoon earlier, so that she could just go on a trip without having to make all of the arrangements and deal with ticketing. She had done an awful lot of it this summer with the wedding, and all of our various travels, and was tired of leading on it. Despite this, here we were, me sitting by and her dealing with all of the ins and outs of a fairly complex trip, but I could not help it. Jumping around different screens with the cruise agent while deciding decks and cabins, and all of that, would have been a challenge for me and I was not good with that kind of stress. When she got done, she came over to me and hugged me out of delight that we were going away together—just the two of us. I was thrilled too. We would have our own time and visiting Halifax and other points of interest in Canada would be a great trip. As she hugged me she said, "Why do I have to do all of the arranging?"

"Because I am paying for it" I responded.

I was immediately aware that this was a really lousy thing for me to say on several levels. I realized this as soon as it came out of my mouth, but it was already out, and I knew she would be upset by it. Whatever money we had was ours, not mine, and I needed to help with details more, as she had requested. She pulled back and looked at me. I apologized and corrected that it was "our" money, and the moment passed quickly in the excitement. But I needed to change this habit of thought. We did not have an agreement where I paid and she did all the work of travel agency, and yet that's the pattern we fell into. We both worked, and although I needed her to do much of the detail work, especially on screen, I *could* do more of it that I was passing off to her. I would need to rethink my behavior, or risk slipping further into a bad dynamic between my sense of entitlement and her sense of obligation to me.

The relational "deal" issue popped up again shortly after this when Jami and Mike took me out for a late birthday dinner. We sat on the terrace at Lucky 32's on a lovely summer night, ate salads, and caught up on news and relived old inside jokes. There was a point in the conversation where Jami asked me how my eyes were doing, and I explained how my night vision had gotten worse and that Hema was doing most of the night driving now. It had also come up in discussion how she and her mom were cooking wonderful meals every day during their stay. Jami quipped, "Hey can you cook, and drive at night? … Yes … Hey, let's get married!"

We all laughed and it was no doubt meant in good fun—he was making a clever connection between things we had discussed. But I am sure others were trying to figure out what the "deal" of our relationship might be, just as we occasionally did about other couples. Although this was an offhand remark meant to be funny, it was a clue to what he thought our relationship might be about. Hema and I had discussed several times that we would always take care of each other, but we never explicitly discussed any specific agreement or exchange constituting an agreement or "deal." I think both of us would agree that we loved each other first and foremost, and that the give and take was part of how we complemented each other as partners.

One weekend in mid-July, I decided I was going to revive my interest in rock cutting, so I dusted off the rocks I had already cut, and enjoyed handling them and imagining them in jewelry. I set aside a couple of pieces to work on but then got busy with the more immediate daily work of gardening. But I had good intentions to work on some rock cutting projects. I did reorganize things a bit, and categorize my rough rock slabs into "jaspers/agates", "petrified rocks", and "others" in old shoe boxes. It was good to fiddle around with them and imagine getting back into the hobby at some point soon. Perhaps this summer I would surprise Hema with a suit of stones to make a unique necklace for her. It would give me something to aim for. For months now my equipment had sat idle with a cover over it in our cramped little home office. In reality, I could not quite get the plan into motion, and everything continued to sit there until the next time I would think about reviving this hobby. Old hobbies die hard.

I noticed that I had more or less stopped consciously checking my eyes for how well they could see, as I had done habitually a year or so ago. It was a fruitless habit as it was impossible to tell if, and how much, my vision had changed. One morning I was snuggled up behind Hema and found myself looking at the wood window blinds. They offered horizontal lines which could be useful in checking visual acuity because distortions in lines is a good way to tell how much vision had been negatively impacted. I was not closing one then the other to compare them, but I was darting my eyes around and seeing if the new spot I looked at was clear—as if I might beat the blurriness to the next point for a split second before the blurriness could catch up. The game was largely unconscious. I had no idea if I was doing this frequently or not, but I knew I could not really beat the blur, however quickly I darted my eyes around.

I had heard nothing from my brother David about his vision in a long time, so I emailed him to ask how his eyes were doing. I knew he would never initiate the discussion unless there was some specific news to report. After a few days, he wrote back to say that he thought his left eye had improved slightly, but that he would go back for follow-up tests in August. I was pleased that he had not experienced any noticeable decline, but I also wondered if it had improved or if he had simply gotten used to it and adapted to accommodate it. I did not say anything to question his optimism, but I made a note to myself that I would check in with him after his appointment in a month of so for more details.

After Hema's parents left town she developed a plan to change some rooms around again. I was resistant at first, given that the furniture had been that way several years before. I felt like we were on a silly slow rotation that just wasted time and energy. She pressed on anyway and, after spending a day reorganizing, I could appreciate what she was trying to do. It was a much better use of the small space we had. One effect of the move around was that I went through my rough rock cutting material again. This time I reorganized it all into categories and boxes. I also had a good place for the equipment now and committed to trying to cut a stone this summer before going back to school. In early august I still had not done anything yet, but at least I was thinking about it. The old hobby pulled at my creative instincts—especially when I looked at stones I had cut and admired them. I was drawn to the fossilized materials—petrified wood and fossilized coral. I picked out some pieces that I wanted to cut, but actually switching the machine on and finding time to do it were just slightly out of reach. On some level I was resisting the step to get back into cutting stones. Perhaps this way of expressing myself was just slowly slipping away forever and I had a hard time accepting it. I certainly was not ready to get rid of the equipment and rocks, even though we could definitely have used the space that this would have created.

Cruising

On the last day of July we made our way to New York and picked up the ship "Carnival Glory" there. It was a huge ship—a floating resort on the move—cutting quickly through the water on its way north to Canada. It was a great time and, despite some of the daily information being too small to read, I was fine except for one very odd moment. One evening after walking to the 24 hour dining room for some late night tea, we saw a few people by the pool sitting in sun loungers. They were getting ready to watch a film on the big screen by the pool. It was a movie about freeing a family of whales from the Alaskan ice—a movie that Hema had wanted to see for a while. Why not, we thought? It was a lovely evening under the north Atlantic sky and we had never seen an open air movie before. A fresh, cool, starry sky, and a nice story to get lost in for a while were a great combination. After sitting watching the movie for a while we were both getting cold, but especially Hema, who was almost always cold. Her feet were freezing. I volunteered to go back to our rooms just two floors below, and get our nice thick bathrobes so we could watch the movie bundled up in comfort. I moved briskly to the 8th floor—following the path that we had taken several times. I noticed that the décor was an odd mix of Italian and Mexican with an overall dark brown over patterned—busy—style. It was like someone was wearing a paisley and a strip and a different stripe all in the same outfit. This added to the visual confusion of the place for me. Walking down the corridor, I got to where I thought our room was located, but it was not our room. The door should have been the other way round. Suddenly a little anxious, I could not remember the number of our room. I walked up and down the corridor and could not jolt my memory. I started to get a little fearful. I knew I would find it eventually, but I just could not figure out which one was ours. I tried the card in a few doors thinking this was surely our number. Was it 8245 or 8452? I could not remember, and nothing was giving me a clue from walking around. Fortunately no one caught me trying their doors, as that would have been a difficult thing to explain. I was lost on my own floor. After a frustrating few minutes I gave up and went back to find Hema. She laughed as I showed up empty handed—her feet still freezing. She told me the number again and I committed it to memory. She offered to go get the robes but I insisted I would do it. I went back down to the 8th floor and the same thing happened all over again. Something was just not clicking for me. I had no visual clues as to where our room was, as everything looked exactly the same. I walked around again from one end of the floor to the other and, again, had to give up and go find Hema. I was panicking inside, wondering how I would explain this to the person at the front desk, if I had to go to the lobby and ask for help. I would look like an idiot. Again, I gave up and sought the safety of Hema's help. Again, I showed up with no warm robes and, by now, the movie was well under way. She almost insisted on going for them but I could not face that so I had her spell out the number again and just hoped my mind would connect the number to what I was seeing as I looked at the cabin numbers. Somehow this time I recognized the way we would normally go back to our room from the upper deck, and I knew I was close this time. Relief, the key worked. Why could I not remember the room? Was my brain tired from the long day walking around ashore, or my eyes worn out from the day in the bright hot sun, and the evening in a dark brown ship with too many clashing patterns in the decor? Was I unable to see the number and register that it was our room? I never really figured out what happened that night. But I just simply could not see the connection between our room number and the cabins I was looking at. With great relief I made my way back up to the lido deck, and we enjoyed the warm humane story of whales finding their way to safety with the help of kind humans—albeit some of them politically motivated.

At the time, I made no parallel connection between their struggle and mine and the kindness of Hema in guiding me! Had I simply blanked on the instructions I did not listen to carefully enough? Had my brain gone to sleep after a long day ashore? Was there some odd disconnect between my brain and my eyes as they struggled to recognize anything? Or had I come to rely too much on Hema's lead? After all, she did take most of the lead in finding our way around the ship. She knew our way around within a day or so, and I relied on her to know where to go. I was becoming more reliant on her eyes and sense of direction, and this clumsy comical moment looking for our own room was a jolting reminder of this. She had developed body knowledge of how it felt to walk to our room, and I had relied on that without internalizing it for myself, so that I could do it for myself. After this, I purposefully set a few tasks involving coming back and forth to the room to and from other locations on the ship, separately, so I would have to master the route. All of this was odd though, because I could see the cabin numbers clearly and could memorize the cabin number, so why could I not put them together that night?

On the ship we were such a long way away from home, but I knew the new academic year was just around the corner, just a week or two away. I knew I was a little worried—especially about driving home at night and in the early morning when the days got shorted soon. I also knew that even if things remained stable, there was much eye fatigue and classroom challenges up ahead this year. And I was worried about how long I would be able to handle things effectively. Hema's job at the community college was perilously close to being cut due to state budget cutbacks. I felt the slight nag of pressure and worry in the back of my mind as things began to rely on me. I was perilously close to having to struggle to see well, and here we were possibly shifting to rely on my salary and job for health benefits and everything else. At the same time it felt like a good time for Hema to explore new interests, and build towards new possibilities beyond the adjunct faculty member's life of renewable one year contracts. My deep wish was for her to have something she enjoyed, and through which she could sustain herself if anything happened to me. I wanted, more than anything, for her to be happy and safe, and perhaps we needed this short term change to get there for the longer term. Living my life around someone else's needs was new for me, and I was enjoying it—but it was worrying because of my vision issues. But we were determined to go forward with our life together, and make good things happen for both of us.

· 13 ·

STABILITY

Living and Working as Well as I Could

One early morning after we had returned home from the cruise, I went for a walk alone at the park. For some reason my mind focused on being thankful for the ability to drive here and still walk independently. Oddly for me, as I was not a religious person, I began to thank God for my ability to still do something so simple that meant so much to me. My mind slipped back to a song by Rich Mullins from many years ago entitled, "Peace" and I recalled some of the song and sung it with my minds voice as I walked along. However long this period of stability lasted, I was deeply thankful, and that is just how my mind and body felt and expressed the emotion that particular day.

That summer we grew fruits and vegetables as we always did, and we had developed the tradition of trying to grow something new each year. This year it was okra. Watching the beautiful and exotic looking okra flowers bloom, and our paw paw fruits ripen in abundance this year, and seeing Hema taste one for the first time just as I did, was wonderful sensory celebrations of togetherness for us.

Navigating Work Challenges

Amidst this bright and colorful beauty, I began to think about going back to school again. I set myself some technology goals. Specifically, I wanted to use technology in the classroom—something I had not done at all since my eye problems began. I knew I was way behind the times, and had a good ten years left in my career. I needed to do some catching up. On the first night of my graduate class I logged in before class and pulled up a webpage I wanted to share with them. Unfortunately, I had to hold my face right up to the glass case in which the screen was housed as it was a small screen set back in the cabinet. I could not see it without looking around the letters on the screen. I would have felt very self-conscious if I had done this in front of the class. This was essentially the first time I had pulled up a page on screen in class since my eye problems began, and it did not go well.

On the second day of my 11 am class I walked in again and the classroom was stifling. Some rooms were cold, and some were hot, and no one seemed to do anything about it. As I read through the roll, my vision almost fuzzed out again. I could just barely read the names. I know I was slow and I had not told them anything about my eye conditions. I would do that when needed. As my eyes fuzzed out, I could feel the sweat beading and rolling at the bottom of my back and on my chest. I waited for the anxious moment to pass, and pressed on as normal.

At the end of the busy first week we got together with Pat and Michael at Chinese kitchen in Quaker Village. It was an area and route that was familiar to me as I used to live near there, so I was ok driving us there. Hema had just gotten home after a long day and a lot of driving around, so I was glad to step in and do driving duties for the evening. Along the long winding two lane Westridge road across to Friendly Avenue I was fine, although there were moments when I had to tell myself that the car coming towards me was not in my lane. Those were frightening micro-moments but I knew the chances that they were actually in my lane were minimal. Coming home, the rain had begun, and it became more of a scary drive for me. As I began driving, I needed to take a simple right turn onto Friendly Avenue. Nervously I asked Hema for affirmation that I was ok to turn. In the rainy dark, I just needed a little surety. She recognized I was nervous and asked if she could drive. I said I would be ok. She asked me how well I could see, and I had no idea how to quantify an answer for her. She told me to pull over and let her drive. I said I was ok. She repeated the directive and, because I was uptight about driving, I shushed her. I immediately realized this was very harsh. She let the moment go, but I knew I was not being kind. What was I doing shushing my wife when she offered to help me? I did not understand it myself, and I am sure she did not. She was offering to drive us home. As we continued on the 15 min drive home she coached me on where the turns were, and told me I was doing fine a few times. She was so kind, even when I was not. The only part I got nervous about again was where the road went from two to one lane. The road lighting was very patchy. Sometimes there were street lights, and then other sections were completely dark. It was a relief to get home, and I actually thought I would be fine night driving for a while, as long as I knew the road, and there was some external street lighting.

In my graduate class called "Positive Communication Research" as part of my introduction of the class, I told them about my experiences with how people and their talk had impacted my own journey into visual impairment, as I had done in a class visit a semester or two earlier. Some of the same students were in that class and remembered my story. Simply, what people said to me had saved me from despair, and that is why I wanted to study and teach the positive side of communication. I could not put it any more succinctly that that! I had said nothing so far to my other two classes as this issue had not arisen. I was still sharing with classes only when it was relevant to them.

Hema saw something on tv about motion activated closet lights that come on when you open the closet in the dark. She was thinking of me—as it is hard to see in closets when there is no direct light in them. She ordered them and, when they arrived, I had the task of opening them up and putting batteries in them. This dragged on for several days, and I know I was asked several times to get the job done! One Wednesday, during the morning, I took a break from prepping for my evening class and fiddled with the tiny screws until I got them all open and the batteries installed. It was no small feat as the screws over the battery containers were the tiniest I had ever seen, and required me finding a screw driver that I had, apparently, put up in the garden shed last summer. I mentioned this incident to my graduate class under the rubric of one of the chapters we were talking about that night. They asked me how many days I had sat on the job not completing the task. It was several, I admitted. They were in unison in deciding that I had gotten the job done just in time. The following week they asked me how the lights were working out!

Another Check-Up

The morning of Friday the 13th of September it was time for my annual check-up at the optometrist's office. As we both prepared our respective teas and coffees in the kitchen, I was snappy, edgy and nervous about the impending appointment. I snapped at Hema a few times out of stress and fear. She took me to the optometrist without complaint, and planned to drop me off and do some needed shopping for groceries.

Thankfully I was not dilated this time. I was surprised as they usually insisted on doing this. The young woman taking me through the test was quiet at first and then, after a little bit of chat back and forth between us, she began talking about her brother who had just moved up to Boston to study at a music conservatory. Clearly she was proud of him. I asked if she also had musical talent and she said yes, and that her whole family was musical. I said they must have some great family gatherings, and she agreed. As we chatted, she was taking me down through the letter tests. They seemed a little easier than last year. I was steaming up the lenses a little less than last year also. My optometrist was upbeat and friendly. As we talked about the year that had slipped quickly between us, she tested my aptitude again with letter tests and then the archaic looking lenses.

"You are seeing significantly better than last year," she said.

"It feels like I am," I replied.

"That's great!" I added.

"I am a little better than last year's 20/70?" I asked, after a brief pause. I was trying to get some quantification.

"Last year's 20/100 more like!" She replied.

"Wow!" I thought to myself. "I had no idea I was at near 20/100 in my right eye last year."

"What?"

"Yes you're prescription will change and you will need new lenses this time. I am going to push you on it this year as things have changed a bit."

"OK I will Doc." I replied.

I called Hema to come and pick me up. As she made her way from shopping for us to the optometrist office I simply looked out into the parking lot, watching the cars go by on Battleground/Westover. It felt good to know that this period of stability was really taking hold, and that things were even much improved. As she picked me up, I felt bad for being snappy earlier.

Over the summer. I had slipped out of the habit of going to the gym. Art and I worked out hard all last year, and it was good to do something different. Summer involved a lot of yard work, so I did not feel the need to go to the gym to work out. On the first day of fall, coincidentally, I decided to get up and drive myself over there and start the process of getting back into working out at the gym. Art had been out for much of the previous spring with medical issues and surgery, so I decided it was time to go back alone. It was still quite light in the mornings so I felt pretty safe to be driving. As I walked in I immediately saw Chris, and said hi to him. We chatted for a minute, him trying to make a joke out of how long it had been since I was there, and us sharing the normal "how are you?" chat. I noticed one of his eyes was bloodshot, so I asked him if he had just had an injection, and how his treatment was going. It was a Monday morning. He told me that he was in church yesterday, and that it worked out this time such that people saw his eye and they were asking him about it. He paused and said, "Well I guess something good can come of it!"

"Yes I guess so," I replied, probably sounding on the neutral end of supportive as I did not know really what he meant. Did he mean that people were now praying for him? Was he using his experience to speak to his fellow believers in some way that was beneficial to them and their faith? In the quick transient moment entering the gym, I did not ask for clarification, and he was gone to his workout routine. Even not knowing quite what he meant, I was struck by how we were both, in our own and very different ways, trying to make something positive out of the experience—him through hi relationships to God and fellow believers, me through my writing on the subject of vision loss.

The Light and the Dark of Stability

One evening in early October, some students leading the discussion in my graduate class wanted to show a Ted talk or you-tube clip on the topic for the evening. We turned the lights off and enjoyed the clip. When the lights came back on abruptly, I could not see much of anything. I had to pause while I could come back into sightedness. The class quickly adjusted and continued with their discussion. They seamlessly adapted and accommodated, taking over the moment where I was struggling. They were a great group.

When I told them about my eye conditions early in the semester one student, Michael, was kind enough to say "I will drive you home." This was a lovely gesture from a student I had liked as an undergraduate, and who was now back here with us in graduate school. At the same time when people make these kind gestures part of my mind always wondered if they realized how complicated such an arrangement would be, if it were meant literally. Did they realize that I would need to also get here in the first place, and would need at least one or two rides each and every work-day? In other words, the practicality of just a ride home was limited, but kind nonetheless.

On Friday evening, October 4th, Hema insisted that I suggest a place to go for dinner. I rarely lead in this department, preferring her to choose somewhere she would like to go. This time I had to choose. I asked her if she wanted to go back to the restaurant in Burlington where we had our wedding reception in May. Luckily she was thrilled to go back to enjoy a dinner out there. On the way back she wanted some tiramisu from the fresh market, so we stopped by. She had driven all the way there and back to Burlington, so I offered to drive the five minutes home from the fresh market. It was getting dark and, as I waited on a flashing arrow to turn left onto Pisgah church road, I told her that I was having a hard time seeing if I could make it as judging the distance from oncoming traffic was difficult. The cars with headlights on pointing at me waiting to turn left at the intersection were blinding me, and I felt nervous to drive out and take a risk. I told Hema that I hated the new flashing arrows, and preferred to just have a green or red choice. She said that from now on I should not turn left at night across traffic. If I were in this spot again I would drive straight down Lawndale and take a simpler left into the neighborhood that way. I agreed. She went on to tell me that I could also just wait until I got a green light. I replied that if someone were behind me, also wanting to turn left at the intersection, then they would not be understanding of my choice. Rather, they would be honking at me to go when there was an appropriate gap in oncoming traffic. To know that other drivers were annoyed at me or against me in any way would make me more anxious about driving. She indicated that I could now turn left, which I did. As we drove along the road with her precious tiramisu—a road I had driven hundreds of times, I almost missed the right turn.

"Here!" She shouted.

"Oh wow. I almost missed it," I replied—braking too hard, and only just swinging the car right onto Normandy. There was a moment of quiet, and then she said, "Well what's the worst that could happen? We would simply do a U turn and come back, right?!"

"Yes I guess so," I replied, unconvinced that it was so simple. If someone was behind me and I braked like that, it could have been tricky I thought to myself, but said nothing.

In October we celebrated Diwali-the festival of lights, at home with Pat and Michael, and Roy and RuthAnn. Hema had made a special effort by decorating the house with small oil lamps, as well as cooking a wonderful meal. As we all sat around, I jumped up to refresh everybody's wine glasses. As I navigated around the small living room cramped with people and furniture, somehow I did not see several small candles clustered together on the floor. I accidentally kicked them sending wax flying all over the floor around them. It was an embarrassing moment standing there with a bottle of wine and wax everywhere. Nobody said anything, but I apologized and stood there awkwardly wondering if I should try to clean up the wax. I left it, and the evening continued on. I just could not understand why I did not see them. Days later, I knelt on the floor carefully scraping off the wax with a paint scraper.

Art, my workout buddy from last year, began to have prostate issues and he was facing surgery, with all of its scary prospects. As we talked about it one day close to the surgery date, I told him that I understood that it must be a frightening prospect. He replied that he now understood how I must have felt facing my eye problems, and all of its scary prospects. The surgery went well and everything turned out fine, but I knew exactly the fear and dread he had in the lead up to that surgery.

Hema and I decided to go home to see my family for Christmas. We enjoyed seeing everyone, although not all on the same day. David came up to stay with us for a night. During his time there, we talked briefly about the possibility of a genetic aspect of our eye disorders as we are twins. The conversation was brief on the topic, as neither of us knew what we had at the time. We described our conditions differently—mine being Cone Dystrophy, and having blind spots from scars where the retinas swelled. He described his condition as having a hole in each retina, though he had no name for it at this point. We both believed that our respective conditions were stable at the moment. That was the extent of our conversation about our eyes. I wished we would have known more, and I wished we would have opened up a bit more about the experience so far, but we could not get there with the knowledge and vocabulary we had so far.

Paul and his wife Jacky came up the next day after David had gone home. I remember the last time we talked on the phone he prodded me to make sure I got the best treatment that I could. During the course of the evening he asked me how my eyes were doing. I told him they were ok and, empathically for a moment, he responded that he would rather lose his right arm than his eyes. I think everyone would probably say the same thing, but I appreciated it. His wife was still deep in grief for the bizarre loss of their middle son, Paddy. This was unspoken during the time there. Perhaps quiet empathy was a premium on this particular trip, given what they had been through with his mysterious and tragic accidental death. We all had something that needed an understanding touch without necessarily saying much, and we all managed to navigate the evening well.

Oddly, between January and May I put aside issues pertaining to my eyes, believing that we had an explanation, an accurate name, and that everything was stable. Life settled into a comfortable routine as the spring semester raced by. I only remembered a couple of moments that were poignant. One in particular involved me leaving the room during a particularly gruesome moment in a Criminal Minds episode when a victim was having their eyes gouged out by a serial killer. I just could not watch the scene. Also in April, when spring was in full bloom and we were interested in outdoor pursuits for the upcoming summer, we bought ourselves tennis gear. It was Hema's idea and, I thought, if my wife wants to play I will give it a retry. I believed I could see well enough to bat around with her. Oddly again though, we did not play at all that summer.

I made my follow-up appointment for Friday July 11th with Dr. Sanders. Would continuing stability be the theme for that meeting, I hoped and wondered? I was looking forward to it actually, because I believed it would still be good news. Hema said she would go with me and drive me home under what was likely to be a blazing summer sky. If I drove myself home still dilated, the sun would have made we want to scream and wear at least two layers of sunglasses.

During that summer, Dad was slowly but surely being diagnosed with cancer. A set of tests a scan, some waiting, more scans, more tests, more waiting, a different specialist. He was enduring the NHS runaround, but a picture was emerging—bladder cancer. He had a cancer removed from his bladder, and there was possibly a shadow on the liver. His comment about giving me an eye came back amidst the swirl of grief and other emotions. It was obvious that dad was heading for a tough time. Was there something poignantly meaningful I could say to help as he had? What would pop out during our conversations besides "How did the appointment go?"; "Oh dear!" and, "Let's see what they say next time"? Nothing particularly deep or poignant was said by me though. Mostly I just made note of the days when he had appointments and treatments, and I made sure I called to check for updates on the following days.

To celebrate my 52nd birthday we went to a spa near Charlotte. Hema treated me to a mud wrap treatment. It was lovely. We were leaving the spa and had decided to go to the mall to look around. As I was putting my clip-ons in my breast pocket, one of the lenses broke from the flimsy little frames. I panicked angrily. Where would I find a replacement? How could this happen now, here, so far from home? Somehow I got the lens to stay on the glasses and I spend the hour or so in the mall carrying the glasses with the clip-ons attached. I was afraid to take them off the glasses for fear that they would come apart again, but I could not wear the glasses with them on inside the mall—it was too dark. So I shuffled them around in my hand and acted like a

52 year old baby. I was fussy and childish about it—expecting the mindreading focused attention of Hema who was busy trying to make sure I had a nice time. Sometimes she called me her 4 year old, and here I was! I often wondered how much her interest in emotional intelligence was sparked by my lack of it! I usually bought clip-ons at Walgreen's, but there was not one anywhere around. I was moody and, stupidly, resisted embracing the carefree time she had organized for me.

One Saturday afternoon, we took our Nepali friend, Ankita, and her mother, who was visiting from Nepal, to the small zoo and aquarium in Greensboro, just for something to do. She visited to drop off a guitar I lent her, and to hang out for a few hours to say goodbye. She was going to Kansas City to stay with her girl pal after finishing her masters, and then on to stay with relatives in Texas. I knew I would miss her. Somehow I never told her about my eyes, but eased her into the issue through some small moments during this parting get together. We were all singing along to song that she liked, and that we had played together before, and that she wanted us to sing for her mother. I needed her to adjust the zoom on the IPad so that I could see the music and play guitar to the song, which she did—even telling me the chord changes out loud. She began to figure out something was wrong, but did not ask for any further details.

We were all taken with the tiger at the zoo, who walked past us many times. As we approached the tiger compound I got out my binoculars to take a closer look.

"You need binoculars to see that?" She asked, perhaps linking this moment to the music moment just a short while earlier.

"No, I need binoculars to see it up close." I replied, showing her my limitations.

The best picture I took that day in the aquarium was of her blowing a kiss to a penguin who was staring at her just behind the glass she was up close to. I believe the penguin was actually sleeping, with eyes half closed, but we left that out of the suggested narrative of a kiss upon first encounter with a penguin. There was something about her that the camera loved and even I took a decent picture. I posted it to Facebook and many of her Nepali friends liked it.

Although we had adapted well to where I now was at the end of year three there were moments when the control seemed fragile, and I had occasional moments of inner panic and outer anger. Old friends Jami and Mike invited me for a birthday movie a couple of days after my birthday. I chose the movie. There was not much playing. Maybe we could all enjoy Jersey Boys? They preferred the friendly center cinema. I had not driven outside of my comfort zones alone in a long time. As I slowed to take a left turn into the movie parking lot I had a moment of inner panic. Was I at the right cinema? I was turning left, but we usually turn right into the one near home. Strange panic. Had I messed up and driven to the wrong place? I would have to rush to the other one. It was a light summer evening with nothing to worry about, and quickly realized I was at the correct place. But the moment of panic was odd and off-centering.

At the end of the spring semester, I friended Bethany from my class, who had her own retinal disease that we had discussed. I wanted to keep in touch with her about her eyes. Perhaps it would be a point of connection for us. I was hoping to get together with her later in the summer to talk about vision and our common experiences, but she moved to Charlotte. From her posts it looked like she was having a fun summer. Although we did not get together to talk more deeply about our eye experiences, her great sense of humor about everyday things was good for me to see regularly through her posts, as I knew I needed to be more like that. We rarely talked about eye problems directly, but I learned a lot from seeing how she made humor out of the silliness of everyday things.

On Thursday July 10th I started to visualize the trip to Dr. Sander's office the next day. I was buoyed by the fact that Hema would drive me there, so there would be no painful glare issues while driving back home. She also had begun to think about reorganizing life around my eye condition. As she sat on the bed with me on Thursday night, she talked about how her working more from home and quitting her job at GTCC would be better for me anyway. She imagined that she would likely be driving me around, and running around with a baby-if that happened for us in the years to come. She was happy to be visualizing her life helping me and creating a family, and I could not imagine my life without her, or her dreams.

Looking back on the year, I did not spend as much time this year thinking about eye problems. I was busy getting married and adapting to that. Consequently, I did not make any contacts or connections into the world of others with similar problems, which I would have liked to have done. I did not research anything to do with my eye disease. I did not cut any rocks. I did not feel the urgency I did a year or two ago, and I simply got down to living and working as well as I could. I put much of my writing energy into my work on bringing light to the dark topic of dowry conflict in India. Classes went very well, although I know I am sorely lacking in the deft touch of new technology—where were the nifty segues to illustrative you-tube clips?

Where was the spontaneous or even planned downloading of relevant material in class? Where was even a single power point slide? Could I take more chances this year and just hope I could see the small in-class control panels or remote buttons? Could I simply just rely on others in class to do what I could not do, and just get on with it? What was I afraid of? I got great reviews and teaching scores, but I knew my students were increasingly visually oriented. I started to realize that if I did not provide visual stimuli they would find it themselves, cell phones under, and increasingly *on*, their desks. Those of us who teach can probably relate to the he tell-tale finger whoosh of the browse that students go to when their eyes are bored and in search of something, or thumb whirr of being partly here and partly somewhere else simultaneously.

Thinking about my upcoming appointment with Dr. Sanders, I was curious to hear the update from a year ago. Had I declined and just adapted and blocked out the decline? Was it so gradual that—like the poor creature dropped into gradually hotter cooking water—I did not notice what was happening to me? I actually felt that I could see better than a year ago, but only the dreary letter test, flash upon flash of retinal pictures, and the deft insight and supportive words of Dr. Sanders would clarify.

YEAR 4

July 2014–July 2015

· 14 ·

UNANSWERED QUESTIONS— IN SEARCH OF WHAT, WHEN, AND WHY?

"So, did they give you a new eyeball?!" A middle-aged son joked, playfully, as his elderly mother made her way back out into the waiting room after completing her treatment.

"No! He said it all looks perdy good." She replied, with a southern twang, and in a resigned tone.

She then chatted briefly with two other elderly ladies whom she appeared to know. One was here to be treated and the other one was accompanying her, and probably doing the driving. The one accompanying the patient said to the small group around her, "She's got to have a shot."

"Yes in my left eye," the patient clarified.

"She's had one in each before but this time it's just the one." Her friend added—perhaps trying to emphasize the positive.

"Aww I've had so many it don't bother me none n' more." The patient explained, stoically.

I was back once again in the waiting room among my fellow eye patients after a year, happily, without such appointments. I was soaking in the moment, paying attention to everything. To fill in the time a bit, I tried to estimate how long I would be waiting based on who else was there. This looked like a fairly busy morning. An hour and a half at least, was my guess.

It was a rare and lovely cool gray, heavily overcast, Friday in July (11th). These days, a perfect driving day for me. It was the kind of day where I would have been fine driving myself there and back as I had many times before, without battling the bright sun, but Hema insisted—driving me there and staying while I checked in and paid the obligatory co-pay. Then she left and I sat down near an elderly couple, waiting for my turn. As it had been a year since I had been here, I made a point of noticing what was the same and what had changed—just to reconnect with the place. The water feature was switched off, thankfully—I am not sure why but I never liked it. The decorations and magazines were the same—bland and uninteresting to me. I recognized several employees who were still here: the blonde assistant, who had several times given me her little finger to stare at so that my eyes did not move while receiving injections, was here. She looked like she was now managing the consulting rooms—at one point knocking authoritatively on a door and asking to see someone for "a quick word." Clare, the office staff member was not here unfortunately as she had been a constant, if minor, character in my story so far. The small guy with the motility challenges was still here, and I felt good for him—he was keeping a good steady job despite his difficulties. I do not know why I thought about him in this way. Perhaps in some way I was comparing myself to him, in an empathic way, as I too was managing to be productive and relatively successful at work, despite challenges. The pot-bellied guy who takes the retina pictures was also still here—still looking mildly disinterested as he always seemed to be. Two of the technicians who have given me eye tests, drops, and so on, were still here. Everything felt familiar and comfortable.

The patient demographic appeared the same in terms of age range: 50 and above. I had only recently begun to see myself in this demographic. Up to this point I had always imagined that I was the youngest person here, and most of the time I was. An elderly African American lady entered the waiting room from outside, and insisted on saying good morning to all of us together—fellow patients. Most of us managed a muted greeting in return to her somewhat unusual gesture. I checked my watch and I had been here for half an hour already. Things were moving along quite well, and I reevaluated my estimate down a little. Maybe only an hour.

The elderly lady who was completing her treatment when I arrived, left with her son. The other two ladies and I followed each other through the testing and treatment process in close proximity. We became momentary travel friends of sorts—passing time as we passed through. We were friendly without actually having a full or personal conversation, or making a lasting connection. We shared a few knowing nods and chuckles at the shared experiences—it was valuable human affirmation in a difficult and stressful place. While we all waited, their conversations touched on other friends and relatives and their various ongoing treatments. Interspersed with this were comments about how cold the doctor's office was.

"We should have brought blankets!" One quipped after a period of silence as we waited between the eye test room, and the retinal photography room. They were both wearing half-length Capri pants, exposing the bottoms of their legs. I had clothes covering me entirely, and was still cold, so I know they were only half joking about the blankets.

"I could have fallen asleep right here if we had blankets" added the patient, in what appears to be a playful dig, both at the amount of time we wait between stages of the appointment, and the coldness of the office.

I smiled, and we all acknowledged the joke. They were joking just loudly enough to include me.

"Dr. Sanders has them cold hands too!" She added, chaining onto the coldness theme, adding another layer to the humorous moment, and the three of us rose to a chuckle together. Later, after my visit here was done, and I waited in the lobby for Hema to drive here and pick me up, they both walked by to leave the building together.

"Are you still waiting?" One of them joked in my direction, and we all laughed momentarily as we connected on the joke one last time. These were ladies used to waiting, their humor helping them through one more doctor's appointment in one more day—*being patient*.

From this waiting area I could see that the sky had brightened, and it had turned into the worst kind of light for dilated eyes—thinly overcast and very bright diffused summer light just behind the thin cloud. In these conditions the light seemed to come from all angles with no escape, and no central source to avoid. I was glad Hema would be picking me up and driving us home. I *could* make it, but was glad I did not have to.

In an examining room I had been in many times before, we ran through the usual eye test, stinging drops, examinations, pressure test, blasting bright retina photos sending the entire room, including the new "like us on Facebook" sign, pink. After a short wait, I was ushered into a consulting room where the monitors showed beautiful tropical scenes with bright clear sunlight and thatched beach shelters, clearly designed to relax and distract the patients from the worry of what might unfold while here. I had seen these pictures here before and, partly because of photophobia, I found myself thinking that it would be close to torture to actually visit. Could they show pictures of some nice gloomy overcast, but equally exotic and beautiful places—the kind that I, and many of my fellow patients, would actually prefer these days? I wondered if I was the only one of many who tracked through these rooms every day who thought this.

An Awkward Conversation

Dr. Sanders entered, and we greeted. It was good to see him. He quickly and happily announced that he could find no reason to do more injections—which I anticipated, and was a little surprised to even hear him tell me. "All dried up and no swelling," he clarified. All good news. Yet, as he was dictating notes it became clear that the retinas have thinned a little due to the cone dystrophy, and the blood vessels have atrophied. His assistant also noted these observations, as if this were obvious from the pictures she was looking at on her screen. I was puzzled, so I asked what this meant. He explained the vascular process of thinning relating to the demands of the retina for oxygenated blood. The less blood they demand because of the breakdown of cones, the smaller the vessels get. Again, there did not seem to be anything I could do with this information, or about this development, except understand, although such a noticeable shift in one year was alarming to me. How quickly were they thinning? How long would it be before more serious problems crept in as a result of this one? I do not know why, but I did not ask in that moment, and he never voluntarily addressed these issue to clarify them for me.

To prelude the wrap up of our meeting, he stated that he wanted to see me again in a year to monitor things, and emphasized me coming back if anything changed in the mean-time. He smiled warmly to signal the end of the conversation. I interrupted the flow of the wrap-up and asked him for advice—what he thought about me meeting with Dr. John at Wake Forest in Winston-Salem to learn more about the Cone-Dystrophy. He seemed slightly taken aback. He said fine, but emphasized that there would be no therapeutic gain from such a meeting. He spelled this out for me slowly and carefully. He said he would be happy to send my records to them, if I felt more comfortable there, which took me aback a little also. He was misunderstanding me. Perhaps he was thinking that I was unsatisfied with his care—which I was not, or in search of a second opinion, which, in a way, I suppose I was. I was not thinking someone else was going to cure me. I was not saying I did not think he did a great job treating my retinas. He did, although I probably never said as much. But here I was, in the fourth year since this began, and I still knew nothing about the Cone Dystrophy—what caused it, how quickly it was changing, what this would mean for me, or even if I actually had Cone Dystrophy. I clarified that I wanted to come back here but that the Cone Dystrophy is still a mystery to me, and Wake Forest Baptist Eye Center focuses on research, so it might be helpful. Dr. Sanders paused carefully and returned firmly to the moment, stating that it is Cone Dystrophy, and that there is likely a genetic component to it, as if that is all I needed to know. It seemed that he and his assistant were thinking something in unison as, momentarily, they both had the same look on their faces and shared half a glance between them. But I could not quite tell what their glance meant. Were they thinking I was setting off on a wild and pointless goose chase? Did they think I was not accepting their diagnosis? Were they thinking that I was either here with them *or* there with another doctor, while I was thinking that both places could add to my understanding? Was this an awkward scenario that had occurred here before? I did not really know, but it was an uneasy moment, embedded in narrative layers I did not fully understand. The simple truth was I wanted to know more—*WHY*—but I do not think he understood the desire for a clearer story. Even if the disease itself could not be treated, I wanted to know more about what I had, and why I had it. As I walked out of his consulting room, he looked slightly upset and did not take his eyes off the computer screen as I left. It was an awkward way to leave, and I felt bad about it, but I had to know more.

Onward in Search of What, When, and Why?

I came home, had lunch, slept for an hour as my eyes were tired from the tests, then, at Hema's prompting, I called and made an appointment with Dr. John in the first available slot. July 28th 9:30 am Monday morning. Hema would drive, as this was 45 minutes away by highway. She said several times that she was happy to scale back her work life to be able to drive me around to such appointments as I could not do it myself. We were implicitly agreeing to a shared narrative moving forward: She would scale back on her excessive busy-ness of the last few years as an adjunct teacher with my support, and she could be there for me as I sought more understanding of, and perhaps treatment for, my eye disease. It was an agreement that suited both of us, at least for now.

Something from my discussion with Dr. Sanders came back to me again and again in the space between my appointment with him, and my upcoming appointment with Dr. John. His description of how my blood vessels has atrophied, and my retinas had thinned, played again and again in my mind—pulling fears and anxiety back to the surface after a year or so of relative peace. My eyes were deteriorating visibly and irreversibly, even in the space of a year. The lights were dimming slowly but surely, and I had no definitive idea of when and how or, indeed, *why*. Momentarily, I thought forward ten years to the time when I might retire, and when life is supposed to be relaxing. Would mine be so or, by then, would I be robbed of this time of life by the struggles of this disease? If the vessels had atrophied visibly in one year, then how many good years did I have left? Would technology somehow sweep in as the rescuer of the story? These were heavy and deep and, as yet, unanswered questions. Why were the questions that were so central to me, the very ones that people who might be able to help me answer so carefully skirted around? Did they just not know either? Perhaps the "new guy" would be able to clarify. I looked forward with slightly nervous anticipation to the upcoming appointment, and the possibility of new possibilities.

· 15 ·

A NEW DIAGNOSIS AND LEARNING SELF-ADVOCACY

Probably like most men, I find it difficult to respond to "talk to me now" requests—especially while highway driving, where there is often not much visual interest to stimulate a topic. I was also a little tense as we headed towards my appointment at Wake one warm sunny morning, and was not feeling very conversational. But I knew she needed some noise, some energy in the car besides the lulling hum of the AC. I had nothing much to say, so I switched on NPR, which was airing a BBC news show. Someone was talking about running marathons and losing weight. No longer swilling beer at the pub or laying on the couch watching "telly" with a bag of crisps as the interviewer visualized humorously, he had changed his life for the better. Surprising everyone, including himself, he was now a serious runner.

As we mulled the story, an extraordinarily dangerous driver flew past us, swerving just in front of us between us and the car just in front in the inside lane to our right. He was soon riding up on the person ahead of us, and looking to get around them however he could. Instead of blaming Hema for hogging the left lane and contributing to the problem—a pattern of driving I had all but given up on, knowing that she was tired, we directed our momentary anger towards the young guy breezing between us all at high speed. I noted it was just before 9 am, and guessed that he was late for work. We speculated that he may be watching too many action movies, or playing too many video games involving spectacular car chases—middle-aged people making sense of young and foolish behavior. The moment passed quickly, but it did charge her up and we were also soon moving full speed towards Winston-Salem.

Arriving, I was struck by the scale of the place. It was like parking and finding our way around a medium sized airport. Deck levels, zone colors, lists of towers and other buildings from which to figure out directions. Once we spent a couple of visits here it became a place that felt much smaller and caring. People were helpful with directions, and so on. As we checked in and waited for my number to come up, I took a moment to have Hema look around the room with me at all the elderly people. I told her that this is how many older people spend their days, and to make most of her 40's. The scene was a reminder to get on with life's goals before part of the body began to need more and more attention. She was looking for a spot to call her own where she could grade papers while I was in the examination process, when my number was called and I was quickly into the inner space of the building.

Dr. John was a smart young specialist who took the time to explain things to me, and he engaged me in discussing the images of my retinas. I liked him immediately. He even said Hema could come in and sit with us, if I preferred. I explained that she was grading papers and we pressed on with the meeting. As we were looking closely at the side by side pictures of my retinas, he pointed out the damaged part in the middle of my maculae—the fovea. I could see the left eye looked slightly better, less damaged than the right. I was relying on the left eye to make up for the right eye in everyday tasks and knew that if and when the left eye failed me, I was heading for trouble. I stopped him to have him explain to me the scale of the image, as I could tell it was magnified. "Well," he said—making an indication on the screen—"this is a millimeter in terms of the actual area of the eye."

"So the tiny area damaged in the middle is about two millimeters across, including the dark rings around the fovea?" I asked.

"Yes!" He said. "This image is a *big* magnification!"

"Wow!" I responded, struck by the poignancy of how one or two tiny millimeters have had such an impact on my life. Three millimeters or more of such damage, I assumed, would likely be devastating.

After close examination of the images, and a quick color test, he was ready to make a tentative assertion that this was not Cone-Dystrophy at all, but more likely MacTel. As we talked more, all of the evidence began to circle around this possible new diagnosis. He wanted to see David's information the next time I came in, and we wrapped up the meeting by setting a new appointment time-line for three months. As we stood out by the administrator's desk, Shree walked past and I managed to stop him with a "hello Dr. Shree"!

He stopped and recognized me from when we met at Lata and Nand's dinner party. He said simply, "This is a very smart man!" Presumably he meant for making the effort to come in for a second opinion, as he had encouraged me to do many months ago. We exchanged a quick congratulations on his new baby and, after inquiries about our respective wives, he was on to his next meeting.

Moments later, as I was waiting for the secretary to give me the number for the ERG person in Chapel Hill, I got a touch on the shoulder from behind. It was Dr. Shree and Dr. John asking me to follow them to a nearby consulting room. Dr. Shree took charge: "Pete, we don't think this is cone-dystrophy!" He opened.

I felt oddly emotional, almost in tears, and touched by the care they had taken to pull me into a room to reaffirm that Cone Dystrophy was not a diagnosis they were simply going to run with. It did not make sense to me as a diagnosis with the scant knowledge I had gleaned online, so I knew it must have been glaringly obvious to them.

"Yes, I know, that's what Dr. John told me," I responded, almost choking up, but making sure he got the credit from his tenured senior colleague. For the first time I felt that I might be on course to have some definitional clarity as to what was wrong with me. It was a quick meeting, and I cannot recall what else was said, but I left feeling that this mystery was something they would help me with.

When we were done, Dr. John followed me back to the secretary's counter where she had written the number on a post-it note for me. Dr. John asked her if she would help me make the appointment, but she did not appear to want to do more than give me the number. Perhaps that is not her job, I thought. He asked her again, reminding her that she had done this before, but she simply said that here was the number and smiled nicely, but with an undertone of resistance. Perhaps he was just trying to be extra helpful because I knew his colleague? To diffuse the moment, I quickly said that I could call them, and smiled to myself, recognizing that administrative staff here were probably much like ours in academia—quick to know the boundaries of what is expected of them, especially if they had not had a raise in several years. No big deal, I could call, I thought to myself. Dr. John and I said our farewells after firming up that I would be back in three months. He reiterated that nothing was currently active, so three months was fine, and he tapped me on the shoulder warmly and was gone. As I stood there, gathering my documents and checking that I had everything I needed, the administrative staff member asked me, "Are you related to Graham Kellett?" She inquired.

"No," I replied. "Is he from here?" I responded.

"No!" She responded smiling widely.

"No, no I don't think so!" I added politely, not knowing what to say. I quickly gathered my things and I was on my way out to find Hema. She was busy grading speeches and papers in a corner of the waiting room.

Afterwards, for lunch, we met Nand and his sister, who was in town visiting. As we sat there, Nand talked for the first time about his own glaucoma in one eye that causes some distortion. He had never mentioned this before but now we were seeing the same Doctor, and the topic was central for the day. We talked about wavy lines that should be straight, and how the brain adapts in amazing ways. Then, suddenly, he made a joke about actually enjoying the additional curves his visual distortion brought him. Hema and his sister got the joke before I did—both laughing and grinning widely. His wife Lata was slender, so I guessed the appearance of additional curves were a happy side effect for him. We all enjoyed the silly moment. Hema noted the positive side of Nand's take on his vision problems, "Talk about making light of a tough situation!" She said. She was right. What a gem of a guy he was.

I spent most of that evening searching sites related to the new tentative diagnosis. Some sites made me anxious, "MacTel is a blinding condition …" one began, starkly. Some helped calm me down a bit, "The disease takes between 10–30 years to progress …" explained another, leaving room for hope. Would I be lucky and be on the 30 year end of things? Some sites were more comforting and conversational, as if I were asking a question that they answered with good news, "Is there hope? Yes, most people retain some vision …" Searching online sites was a mixed, up and down, feeling. I did this while Hema grinded away—still grading papers and speeches for her summer school class. I had taken up most of the day she really needed for grading as the final grades were due today. As I slept soundly that night, she worked most of the night to finish grades—a scenario that was too common for us. Amidst the ups and downs of the online search, my mind came back to Dr. John's comment that, if it turned out to be MacTel, this was a much better diagnosis than Cone-Dystrophy. I could not really see why, as they both seemed to me to end up in the same place, but this hopeful conversational fragment was something I had to hold onto for now. Things may not be as bad as we thought they were for the past few years.

Overall, I had a feint sense of relief that we were moving closer to some valuable clarity. I felt good about making the effort to get a second opinion. I also felt good about Dr. John and the choice to go to Wake Forest. One evening, I searched through the website of other nearby eye centers and found nothing in the research of the faculty that made me think I should have gone there instead. I did not find anyone locally with a specific research interest in MacTel. Interspersed with these constructive thoughts, I also felt a deep muted panic that, yes, I would most likely be moving towards being blind in both eyes in this lifetime. In the short term, I also knew that it was highly probable that my left eye would at some point catch up with my right eye—mirroring its decline. That would be a dreaded, and transforming, time to come, I knew.

The very next morning I got a Facebook message from the wife of a close college friend, Dez Malandain, to say that he had died on Sunday, and that his funeral was on Tuesday at the nearby crematorium in Sheffield, England. I was stunned. Poor bugger, I thought. He had just retired. The thought struck me of how fragile and temporary all of us really are, and how little we thought this thought back in the college days together. I thought of contacting Joe, a friend who would remember Dez well from those College days, but I had not heard from him much since he and his wife retired to Flagstaff more than a year ago. He responded with a one line email in March when we sent him a birthday card, but since he retired he has not asked how I was doing once, and the friendship was disappearing to a memory, as Dez had just done. How fragile friendships can be also, even ones of thirty years that you think will last a life time.

I wanted to go for a walk alone, but Hema wanted to come and get some exercise and fresh air. Between the heaviness of the new diagnosis, the death of my college friend I had just found out about, and the fact that Hema was, even now, still not done with grades and this was dragging on *again*, I was irritated and it came out as we argued much of the way, mostly about which path through the park to take. She was exhausted and stressed too, so it was just the bad timing of many things clashing. I wanted a peaceful walk and here we were unloading frustrations and stress on each other. By the end of the loop the air had cleared a bit, but the tense heaviness that clung on was the last thing either of us needed today.

On Thursday of that week, I sent Dr. Shree a quick email thanking him for connecting me with Dr. John, and for stopping by to talk to me. I told him that it was a great experience at the eye center. Within minutes he emailed back for a number at which to reach me. I sent him my number, and within a minute he called me. It was an odd conversation mostly because, for much of it, I did not know what he was driving at. He was trying to suggest something without stating it, perhaps thinking that I would figure it out and say it myself. But I am not familiar enough with the conversational archetypes of his medical world to know what the script was about until he finally spelled it out for me, towards the end of the conversation. After the brief initial greeting, he led: "How did your life change as a result of the diagnosis?"

"Well, I have adjusted to reading on an IPad ..." I replied, trying to figure out where he was going with the topic.

"No! Did you reorganize your life after the diagnosis?" He tried another way at the topic, but I still wasn't sure what he was getting at.

"Not really, I have adapted over the three years ok. It was a shock at first, but I have gotten used to it." I stumbled around for an answer he might be looking for.

"Did your life change as a result of the diagnosis? For example if I got a diagnosis that I had testicular cancer, it would have an impact on my life." He said, more forcefully.

He was helping me with a graphic analogy, and I was starting to get a sense of what he was driving at. Yes it was a terrible shock, and it had an impact on me emotionally for a year or so, but I did not think it was the diagnosis of that specific problem so much as having a retina disease.

"No No! I can't say that it changed my life any more than this diagnosis would have." I said, now aligning more closely with his veiled intent.

"OK!" He sounded like he was about to be much more direct as I was not getting it. "You might be eligible for some financial compensation because you received a wrong diagnosis!"

Ahaaa! I thought to myself. Now I got what he was trying to tell me, although he never quite said it. Wow I thought, *sue Dr. Sanders?* That was the last thing I would have thought of. He had done a great job with the treatment of the edemas, and I liked him enormously. I could not imagine recasting him as a villain or fool, and I could not imagine suing him.

"NO! No" I reiterated, "I don't think that diagnosis really meant that I *reorganized* my life."

Truthfully, I think I would have reacted similarly to either diagnosis based on what I read online. I had so little information, except from online sources, that I never really grasped the magnitude of the original diagnosis. Nor is it obvious from online sources why MacTel is a better diagnosis than Cone

Dystrophy. Dr. Sanders never really said much about it other than that it was not treatable, and that it appeared stable. So, for me, the name of the condition did not affect me as much as the fact that I had a potentially blinding condition. Everything I read online on Cone Dystrophy and MacTel appeared to be quite similar in outcomes: Loss of central vision and possibly, eventually, blindness. Obviously these guys saw them quite differently. The conversation continued: "Well everything I have read suggests both conditions end up essentially in the same place." I said.

"No! This is *much* better. You're going to be ok. I think we can treat this." Shree responded.

"Oh really? ok great." I said.

"Ok it sound like you have that covered then. I will keep an eye on this. We'll talk. Did you get your test done?" He was wrapping up.

"No but I have the number to set up the EEG." I said, a little uncomfortable that I had not called them already—something Hema reminded me of also by Thursday.

"*E*RG!" He corrected.

"Oh ok, ERG. I will call." I assured.

"Ok set that up. We'll talk soon. Bye." He was gone.

Learning Self-Advocacy

The next day it struck me how flatly and passively I had behaved in the early stages of the diagnosis. Why had I not insisted on a second opinion at a credible research institute? Why had I not pushed Dr. Sanders to explain the connection between the alleged Dystrophy and the edemas and other issues manifesting in my eyes which did not make sense? He had separated them, treating what he could, and did not really do much about what he thought was the dystrophy part, or think about how they interrelated. Looking back, I remember him carefully specifying that he was treating the swelling and edemas and not the Dystrophy. I had simply gone along with it, and lived with the lack of a coherent narrative tying the problems together. After all, he seemed consistent with the online information in stating that there was no known treatment or cure for Cone Dystrophy. Looking back on the last few years, I realized I had floated along not really knowing what I had. But I still did not think the misdiagnosis affected my current visual acuity. How a different diagnosis would have affected me psychologically and emotionally I could only guess.

Thursday evening we met Lata, Nand, and his sister, on Tate Street for tea and frozen yogurt after they had dinner. I relived the conversation for Lata that I had with Shree and, as she was also from the medical world, she knew before the punchline what Shree was getting at. Hema believed the wrong diagnosis *had* affected me profoundly. She recounted for the group how I had tried to push her away. "Why would you want to be with a guy who is going to be blind?" She performed my apparently overly dramatic lines from a couple of years ago. I did not remember such a conversation, but she did. She always did! She also hinted that the diagnosis had been central to my reluctance to have children, although for me it was much more about my age and priorities. Lata clarified that this *is* what Shree meant—that my life decisions had been affected by the wrong diagnosis. I had made choices and adjusted my life based on a wrong diagnosis. Again, I said, I did not think the name of the diagnosis specifically was as important to how I reacted so much as having a potentially blinding condition, irrespective of the name. After all, both were classified as maculopathy. It was an interesting semantic issue, but I sat there, again, unable to imagine suing Dr. Sanders.

On reflection, he could have looked a little closer into the possibility of MacTel. He could also have sent me to someone for a second opinion, and an ERG—standard procedures for my new team. But he did not, and here I was, probably no different in terms of current visual ability either way.

In conversations that night with Hema I said I did not want to get involved with lawsuits, and that, perhaps, there was something going on between these doctors and their respective clinics that I did not want to get in the middle of. I noted that Dr. Sanders' new partner used to be with the Wake Forest department. The prompting of a friend on the phone to consider a lawsuit and that it might mean, "$50K that doesn't come out of his pocket directly anyway" left me wondering how anyone wins with such a mentality, and I was more resolved to move on in a constructive way with things.

Important Moments of Learning

The next day I spent an hour or two in a phone-a-thon-run-around. I called the place where I was to get the ERG done at UNC Chapel-Hill, and was told I needed a referral faxed to them. I also needed to specify which of the two tests I needed. I called my ophthalmologist's office and was asked whose attention the fax should go to. I did not know that information either. They could not tell me which test I needed, but would be sure to find out and write it on there when the fax was sent. I logged into my Wake Forest patient portal to make the referral request in writing so it would definitely get done. It would not accept the last four digits of my social security number to log in for the first time. I had to call their tech services who gave me the numbers 9999 to type in until my own number was "in the system." So, after all this time on hold and "select 3 for appointment information," I had made the request, but still did not know anything specific, and it would all have to wait until next week. It was frustrating, but it summed up my lack of patient self-advocacy skills to this point.

Looking back on how I had handled the recent sequence of tasks, I note that I had not written down which type of test I needed, though I remember Dr. John telling me. I had not written down the doctor's name so that the referral would go to the right person. And I had not checked that a referral was being sent to that office so that I could make the appointment. I was still grinding my way up the learning curve as a patient, making mistakes and creating more work for myself—and for Hema. I was wasting time on hold—following labyrinths of keypad decisions to get to the person I needed for each bit of information, to get the next bit of information, to get the appointment I needed. I did not even know if my insurance was covering the appointment I just had, and I began to worry about receiving a large bill. In the end, to my relief, it did cover it all except the copay.

I messaged my brother David, to tell him of the new diagnosis, thinking that it might be relevant to him. At this point he had also been diagnosed with holes in his retinas, but it was as yet, nameless. He was awaiting more consultations in order to reach a specific diagnosis. I asked him if he could request records from his ophthalmologist to help Dr. John figure things out from this end. He responded saying he would look up the name of the condition and thanks. He never mentioned the records part of my request and, even when I followed up again with a request at least for the contact info for his ophthalmologist, he ignored the request. So much for the possibility of a shared collaborative moment! Hema used the lack of his response to revisit her desire that my brothers and I should have more regular phone call contact. We rarely talked on the phone, whereas she talked frequently, almost daily, with her sisters who were all close. She argued that such a request for personal medical information would be much easier if we had a closer ongoing talking relationship. I disagreed with the idea, holding that he would have ignored it even if we were on the phone regularly. She may have been right though. I do not know who was right or wrong on the topic, but he never responded to the request. Perhaps he was looking into it without mentioning it in message chats? Perhaps he did not want another medical issue to deal with after two bouts with cancer in his lifetime so far. Perhaps he just did not want to be that helpful. I had no clear idea.

On our beach trip, pre-semester getaway, to Ocean Isle in early August, Hema drove all the way, despite my offers to share driving. It was bright and hot and she had eye fatigue and headaches from it by the time we got there, after four hours of driving. On the trip there was much tension as we made a couple of wrong turns. Hema was driving and navigating on her IPhone at the same time. She complained that she had to do everything related to the trip: Book the room, drive, and navigate. I complained back at her that she did not engage me with the directions and that, if they were written out for me and, if we had a discussion of the route before-hand, I could help more. I would have a better sense of what towns to look for, and where turns would be coming. Truthfully, I had gotten lazy in helping. I got angry and shouted that I could not read the directions on my IPhone. She heard me, and I heard her, but we were both frustrated, it was hot, and there was a long way to go. I needed to help her. Why should she do everything just because it was a bit of a struggle for me to read things—especially on small screens while wearing my sunglasses? Why did I assume I would simply go on a trip like this with everything planned and organized? Was I assuming that because I paid for the room, and the gas, then she would do all the rest? I realized that this probably was not fair. My money was now ours, and so the tasks associated with travel should also be shared. Before the trip, I could book the room though, and make plans more effectively in future by searching the route and writing it down myself. I remember asking her please could we sit down before a trip and go over the route so I could help avoid wrong turns that added time to the drive? It was a tense start to the trip.

We stayed inside in the afternoons as it was too bright for me, and too hot and sunny for her outside. The window cooler unit struggled to cool the room, and the room quickly became claustrophobic and hot for both of us. Our confinement in the small motel room-like condo caused some tensions, snappiness, and restlessness between us. I grumbled when she wanted to go to Myrtle Beach for fun in the mid afternoon sun on the next to last day we were there. We did go, and ended up having fun on the rides. We zip-lined across a lake which she pushed me to do, despite me not wanting to. The sun was hot and bright for both of us though, and we were ready to come home that night.

We left a day early, recognizing that the bright hot sun of the beach was not for either of us. Seeing people lying in the sun, baking their skins, just seemed so odd to us. I needed to avoid bright sun in my eyes, and she dreaded the quick darkening of her skin that would happen when we were out in the sun walking on the beach. We did not criticize or make fun of anyone, we just realized together, I think, that the beach was a place we would enjoy in the winter. Then we could avoid hot sun, but still enjoy the restorative and restful presence of the ocean on the beach—walking, collecting shells, and so on. On our return she got headaches, again, from the brightness of driving and this lead to a discussion about her sunglasses. They were relatively cheap gray tinted lenses, and not polarized. I could have lent her mine so easily. I felt bad as she drove all the way again. I spent some time that evening searching online for driving glasses for her, and asked her to look at some designs. She was reluctant to spend the money for really good glasses, which made me feel even worse. I would surprise her with some, and resolved to do more of the driving in future. I could easily drive on highways if she directed me—as she would see signs and landmarks much earlier than I did. The eye fatigue, and her struggle with brightness, was a moment of opportunity for empathy—but I could not think of how to say that I experience the same things without it sounding like a competitive or selfish comment. So I left it unsaid, and quietly ordered her some high quality sunglasses, like mine.

The next day, in the afternoon, she wanted me to go to Elon with her to sign her contract to work there as an adjunct teacher in the fall. She was excited to teach at a new place but did not want to drive there alone. The last thing either of us wanted to do was get back in a car today, but she had to sign the document. I did not want to go but, as she showered, I surprised her and got ready and went with her. It was a small gesture to say that I was being supportive and responsive to her requests, and to recognize how much she had driven us around in the last few days. As we walked around the well-manicured campus, and looked around her new building, I could tell she was excited and relieved to be free from the community college environment. She had endured it for three years—paying off debts and contributing to our life together. I wanted her to be happy. I wanted her to enjoy walking across the little street next to campus to the quaint coffee shop to enjoy some time with new colleagues. I wanted her to find things she enjoyed, and wanted to do, while she was here. It was a temporary job, but a much needed change for her.

The new diagnosis, which was apparently a better one, sparked a renewed conversation, albeit mostly one sided, between Hema and me on the topic of having a child. According to Hema, now that my diagnosis was much better, I no longer should operate in the fear of being blind. According to her, this was one of the main reasons I was reluctant to start a family with her. The truth was, everything I read also listed this as a potentially blinding disease. And I did not have the heart to tell Hema that it might also be debilitating as well as hereditary. If we had a child they may suffer this journey too. She uploaded an ovulation calendar and was pressing forward with the plans anyway. I knew she enjoyed the thought of having a baby, so I left the topic alone as much as possible.

Tragically, Robin William's took his own life, it was thought, brought on by depression as a result of his diagnosis of Parkinson's disease. The encouraging words of his wife hit home as I look back on the darker times of my own journey so far. The feelings of despair and fear were powerful at times, and I could understand how a degenerative disease that robs one of faculties so close to one's identity and passions might bring on this level of despair. His wife Susan Schneider said, "It is our hope in the wake of Robin's tragic passing that others will find the strength to seek the care and support they need to treat whatever battles they are facing so they may feel less afraid." (Tara Culp-Ressler, "What Robin Williams' Parkinson's diagnosis teaches us about depression." Think Progress, August 14, 2014). She was right—feeling supported does have an impact on fear levels and, perhaps, fear does impact depressive thoughts, maybe even suicidal thoughts.

A Moment of Sharing with Students

In my 9:30 am class on the first day in August, a student spoke of a conflict with her father over her need for eye surgery. She had contacted me over the summer to prelude her possible need to be out of town for this procedure, so I immediately knew this was her. After my class I found myself talking with her and another student, who also has a serious eye condition. Hayley had contacted me over the break to tell me she might need surgery in Miami, and might miss the first part of the semester. The other student, Melissa, joined us as we chatted, and she shared some of her story of surgery, her fears, and her sense of shock at having a condition that very old people usually have. I could identify, often finding myself being the youngest person sitting in the waiting room. We compared condition names, although I still could not say mine completely, and shared some of the main symptoms and impacts on our vision. Hayley had a condition in which the actual shape of the eye changes, leading to difficulty with vision clarity. Melissa had a different condition in which she struggle with other issues. One has her IPad on dimmest setting. I have mine n the highest brightness. None of us see well at night. And so, we compared, and empathized, after the first class. It was a really nice moment.

Hayley went on to speak of a current conflict with her father who wants her to finish the semester before she has surgery, while she wants to go ahead and do it and risk having to withdraw for a semester. I did not know the background issues of her situation but Melissa and I urged her to go ahead as soon as possible as lost sight is almost always gone forever. We all knew that. People who do not have conditions like ours would probably not fully understand. We all agreed on this point. The conversation between the three of us focused on her situation for a while, as she was right at the point of needing to get something done. Melissa asked how much it would cost, and Hayley said about $5K. There was no one nearer than Miami who could do the surgery, at least as a familiar procedure. We all spoke directly, and sometimes indirectly, of the fear and shock of having serious eye conditions. I asked them if they could still drive and Hayley said she had lots of friends here who can drive her anywhere. I thought to myself, how quickly that can change after college. I did not say anything. Interestingly we all had conditions that had, at this point, impacted one eye much more than the other. At the end of the conversation one of us said what a blessing it is to have two eyes. We all agreed on the marvel of this redundancy and moved on our separate ways to the next class.

Later, I scanned my mind for how to help Hayley. It stayed with me. She seemed to have oriented well to where she was, but you never know with such situations. She had only been diagnosed with a disease for a few months, meaning this was probably an aggressive condition. I knew first-hand that despair was never far away, when the reality of a degenerative condition hits you. This knowledge was, of course, heightened poignantly by the Robin Williams case. I thought how valuable it might be for both of them to journal their experiences, if they were not already, and I made a point of telling myself to tell them in person soon. It was late August—the high point of the "bucket challenge" craze for ALS, and the videos on Facebook were becoming drearily predictable, at least to me. I wondered where all the hoopla was for people with eye disease like these two young women.

At the end of August I still had not gotten my ERG organized and, somehow, the parts were not coming together well. I would have to follow up on Monday again with Wake Forest. I needed to get this organized and I did not want to call Chapel Hill again without sounding like I knew what I was doing.

On Thursday morning in the second week of classes I asked Hayley, just before class, if she was journaling her experience. She smiled and said that, yes she was, and that it helped a lot to write down the experiences. We agreed, connecting briefly around the benefits of writing down funny moments as well as fears. The student next to her asked if she had missed something related to class and we both said no, and I clarified that it was something just between us.

On Thursday morning in the third week of class Hayley told me after class that she will not be here for the upcoming test and asked if we could reschedule for her, which was fine with me. I asked her if she was doing the surgery and she said yes. I was pleased for her and joked that finally her dad agreed. As she walked away towards my office door she joked back, "He had no choice!"

We both laughed. She was taking charge of her health care, and it was good that she was.

The next day Hema checked in with me on the Chapel-Hill ERG appointment process which was, by now, annoying for both of us. She told me to make it a priority to get the appointment sorted out, and that I might need to send them another reminder. He probably forgot, as she said.

An ERG Experience and Beyond

On the morning of Wednesday September 16th I had just picked up my phone from the table to go for a quick morning walk, when it came alive in my hand. It was in silent mode, so it buzzed and lit up. It was a 919 number, which is from the Raleigh area. My instinct was to ignore the call, assuming it to be someone calling for heating and air conditioning work, or automated call from Google, but Hema insisted that I answer it. It was the Ketner Eye Center at UNC, calling to schedule my ERG. I joked with her that I was wondering what had happened to the referral process, and she laughed. I was about to try to track this down again and was not looking forward to the process. The caller was engaging and helpful, and scheduled me neatly on a Friday late morning on October 24th. We would do the exam, have lunch in Chapel hill together, and be home in time for Diwali celebrations, which would begin that Friday October 24th Perfect!

Alie and I completed our first draft of the book chapter on Melissa's story of being a blind professor that we were working on. All of us who wrote chapters for the book were sent a copy of a chapter by a faculty member whose story centered on whether to tell his students that he had recently experienced brain damage. Stricken with a form of aphasia, he had problems recalling vocabulary which is quite central to being an effective professor. His story touched me. Our paper played with the same existential and communicative dilemma—how to be true to oneself and yet clear about being different—impaired in ways that students might not understand or care about. It seemed to be a common theme to both chapters.

We made our way to Chapel Hill, and I was deeply thankful that Hema took charge of the drive there. The clinic was miles from where I pictured it to be, even after looking at the directions map online. I would have been lost, and I would have missed my appointment if I had driven alone.

As we waited in the seated area by the elevators and rest rooms, an elderly man pulling a roller bag stopped outside the men's room just near us. He knocked politely as if it were occupied and, after a brief pause, pushed the door slightly to see if it would open. It was a heavy door and, although not locked, it did not move easily, and he simply gave up—bewildered by it all and unsure of whether it was occupied or not. We felt so sad for him and tried to tell him to push the door harder and go in, as the outside door he was at was only the main entrance and not locked by an occupant, but he was gone round the corner so quickly I do not think he saw or heard us. The assistant came out a few minutes later calling out a name several times to no avail. Perhaps it was him—having wandered off somewhere out of range.

I asked the technician doing my test if I could speak to the Doctor who would interpret my results. The technician disappeared for a while and then came back to say that the doctor would see me today, but that I would have to go back through check-in to register as having as an appointment. She stopped short of saying "so you can be billed for it." I could not believe it. I thought I *had* an appointment! But apparently my appointment only covered the test, not any discussion of the results—no consultation. She did say that she had passed on my information to the Doctor and she found it "interesting." I said thanks and that it was ok—I would not make an appointment, but would talk over the results with Dr. John next week. She could not even come out to see me for a two minute chat I thought to myself-wow! Later that evening my friend John Nostrand listened to the story and simply rubbed his thumb and forefinger together, as if to say, "It's all about the money." Perhaps it was also about insurance coverage too, and the ever present loom of lawsuits for anything said or done that was off scripted protocol. I did not know. I just wanted to tell her about my brother's diagnosis as background information as she examined my ERG results. Perhaps it was not necessary, but it did bother me for a while.

Dr. John said he would send my old ophthalmologist, Dr. Sanders a letter explaining what has been happening, and stressed his desire for the same courtesies if it were him. Dr. John was kind enough to call with the news that the ERG was normal, which essentially ruled out Cone-Dystrophy. I was not sure how this was related, but apparently it was. He also said that his department head had contacted the Eye institute of America with the news that a pair of twins with MacTel existed. I was excited that we might make some even small contribution to research, but I did not hear anything further on this.

At the end of that week, I had my regular prescription eye test. I was thrilled that they said I would not need to be dilated again. That would have been three times in one week, and it was another bright and hot day. My eyes were very tired already from the two other examinations, and from reading a mountain of papers I had to grade. Another piece of good news—my acuity had not changed, so my prescription stayed the same as it was a year ago. That evening. Hema and I had a conversation about struggling to see as a faculty member. We agreed, rightly or not, that many of our students would not understand if it meant delays in getting papers back, and so on. "Do something else"! She imitated them being indifferent and selfish—and the thought worried me. Some would understand and adapt, I convinced myself. They will not, she said, unless they have been through something similar themselves. Hypothetical discussions aside, I was just glad to get through this week, and deeply relieved to have no discernible signs of decline in the past year.

· 16 ·

DISEASE AS RELATIONAL AND FAMILY NARRATIVES

"… I hope this doesn't sound bad, but we *really* want your blood!"
—Jennifer Trombley, Personal Communication (February 13th, 2015)

In the middle of November, I tracked down Mr. Lloyd, my usual visa photographer. I needed him to take pictures for my UK Passport renewal which was due in mid-December. He had given up his studio and was working out of his home which, fortunately, was close by. I found my own way there. As we chatted in his front room studio, the topic came around to him and his wife renewing their driver's licenses. They both dreaded the eye test but he made it through with no problems this time. His wife was more nervous. I could certainly relate to her fear. My own renewal test was due in just 6 short months, and it felt like a crossroads moment looming for me. Our conversation brought back the fears a little. He told me of an elderly man ahead of him in line, and how he felt bad as the employee was reading him his long list of restrictions. We joked that he could basically drive to his mailbox during daylight hours. But, underneath the jokes, my own fears were not far away. I told Mr. Lloyd that even that one little bit of driving freedom probably meant a lot to the old guy. He agreed, and we moved on to other topics, but it brought back fears for me. Would they give me a little time to focus as they did at the eye doctors? Would I get someone who was understanding and reasonable for that one key moment?

Getting Involved

In Chicago in mid-November at our National conference (NCA), I had decided to get involved in the two divisions where my current interests fit best—Peace and Conflict Communication and the Disability Issues Caucus. The Peace and conflict communication session was good. Several of the attendees were writing chapters for my upcoming edited books, and others I had seen before and knew. I was very much at home. Immediately after this, I attended the Disability Caucus business meeting. It was a small group consisting predominantly of disabled attendees. I could not take my eyes off a colleague in front of me over to the right. He had no arms or legs. Propped up in a special wheelchair, he worked on his cell phone with his tongue. He adjusted his glasses periodically by pushing the glasses up against a plastic cup that was clipped into his chair to his left. He sipped on the straw periodically. I was fascinated and saddened at the same time—even, to be honest, slightly repulsed by his reliance on his tongue, which saddened me even more. What a journey each day must be for him. Who took care of him? How did he function as a professor or grad student—whatever he did? How did he function just as a human body moving around and doing the obvious things that arms and legs enable? I had no idea, and could not imagine a day in the life of someone with no arms or legs.

The meeting was dominated by a discussion of the accessibility issues of this hotel and conference. It was a tough venue for disabled people. Small and slow elevators with dimly lit floor indicators, and confusing routes between the conference rooms on different floors, added to the sense that this hotel predated design accommodations for disabled people. It did not help that there were cramped and claustrophobic corridors up on the fourth floor section. People in wheelchairs had a hard time slipping between the water dispensers, and clusters of people waiting for their rooms to come open, where they would be presenting or attending panels. It was reported with much collective joy that next year we would be at the Rio in Las Vegas where all conference facilities and rooms would be on one floor together, and that they were state of the art in terms of accessibility.

I was handed a small pile of meeting minutes to pass back behind me after I took one. The person right behind me was blind. I froze, not knowing whether to give him one or not. What should I do? Obviously it was no use to him, but I also felt awkward passing over him. A person to the back of the room indicated quickly that they already had copies, so I just placed the sheets down next to me, relieved that the uncomfortable moment had passed. Perhaps it was having two business meetings in a row with much of the same information being shared at both. Perhaps it was seeing the people around me who I identified with, but also desperately did not want to become like, but this existential split made me feel an overwhelming urge to leave.

One person began to dominate the discussion with a review of news from the legislative assembly meeting he had attended on behalf of the caucus. I had heard most of the same notes in the Peace and Conflict meeting right before this one. It sounded like all of the business meetings were chewing over the recent case pertaining to a professor who was hired at the University of Illinois, and then had his contract nullified for tweeting something they did not like. I wanted out. Waiting for an opportune moment, I got up and quickly walked directly out of the back door. Outside a blind young man was fiddling with his audio device, I think it was a phone. I silently wished he would be alright, and that he would make it back to his room ok, as I headed back towards mine, and to see Hema.

A Twinned Narrative

Over Thanksgiving weekend my brother David posted to Facebook, "I have just graduated to a giant print Bible-due to vision problems, and of course, nothing to do with age!"

He was obviously feeling the pinch in some things in everyday life. Certainly it sounded like reading regular print was becoming a problem. Perhaps driving and other activities were getting difficult as well. He had not told me much about what was happening. I did not know how to respond. Our supportive comments were sporadic and clipped into short back and forth Facebook messages. No one else had commented or "liked" his post, and it just sort of hung out there uncomfortably. He is sensitive and easily takes things the wrong way, so I thought about it for a while and replied blandly but helpfully, "IPad makes reading a lot easier." The interaction ended there.

He may have gotten some inquiries as his posting may have invited questions, I do not know, but clearly he was noticing some of the same difficulties creeping in through the grey blank spots in his central vision, as I was. Facebook never seemed like the place for things of a problematic and personal nature. Here his post was surrounded by pictures of cats in curious and cute sleeping poses, and political commentaries after the recent Ferguson Missouri grand jury ruling. The warmly affirming, and the harshly polarized, worked better on Facebook than the awkwardly personal.

This year Hema handled everything to do with holiday decorating, including putting up the tree. Something that a year or two ago was so poignant for me now faded into the background. My dad's ongoing battle with bladder cancer was also a factor keeping me not so excited about the festivities this year.

I joined the MacTel group on Facebook—a patient run support site for anyone related to MacTel, but did not really jump in to communicating with anyone or reading posts for now. I was busy trying to get a book chapter finished that I had promised by the end of December, but had not completed yet. The new semester was also center stage, and I worked on syllabi for the classes that were about to begin in just a few days (January 12th).

One night just after Christmas, as I lay in bed about to fall asleep, the bright silvery gray morphing shape appeared again before my closed eyes. I had not noticed it in a long time. It was a heart shape that morphed into two hearts within the bigger heart, then back into one bigger heart shape. My minds eyes followed it closely, ever-changing, as I drifted off to sleep. My friend Sidra had just gotten engaged to be married to Imran. I was pleased for her. Perhaps there was a connection between her good news and the beautiful images my retinas and brain were seeing in the dark?

I had been meaning to contact my brother David for a while, to see if he would be open to participating in some genetic related study. I knew he had not been formally and finally diagnosed and then, out of the blue—perhaps being one more twin moment of synchronicity, I received this message on January 8th 2015:

Pete

"I had another set of eye tests today—confirmed diagnosis of Macular Telangiectasia MacTel. The consultant is part of a global research team (incl USA) and they would be interested in including us and our family-especially with the twin dimension. They could fly you to a USA center (e.g. LA) for a blood sample-or check if there is somewhere nearer (obviously they will pay travel). Would you be up for that? Sounds worthwhile."

I responded quickly, "Hi David yes I had been meaning to pursue this also through the MacTel Project definitely worth exploring the genetics. Who was your consultant? My opth team is a research university also so they could handle it. Otherwise closest center is in Miami."

After reading David's message to Hema, who was distracted by an interesting case of childhood tantrums that were devastating a family on Dr. Phil at the time, I immediately looked up the likely person he saw at Moorfield's Hospital on the MacTel map of participating sites. It was Cathy Egan, but as excited as I was to see something happen, I resolved to wait to hear back from David on exactly who he saw, and how they thought we might best proceed from here. Almost immediately I thought of updating my original ophthalmologist—Dr. Sanders, as I thought he would want to know. But, again, I needed to wait to see this unfold a little first. Most likely I would have Dr. John handle any samples that needed taking, and any connection with the Doctors that was required. My mind was flipping through the possibilities and logistics of how we would participate in the study. I went online again and found Dr. Gillies updating that 24 families had been identified as having siblings with the condition. Perhaps, somewhere out there, were other twins with MacTel I could talk to. Perhaps we would be the first twins to participate in the study. I was excited that something good might come of this. Then, the gentle irony of perhaps at some point providing good data for someone for their research slipped into mind and brought a grin to my face—I was always on the lookout for good data myself for my own research.

The next morning was frosty and bright. I waited for the bug guy to show up to spray around outside the house. I sent Dr. Egan an email to state that we would both be thrilled to participate as subjects in the MacTel project in any way we could. I originally wrote "willing": but changed it to "thrilled" before I sent the email. I messaged David to tell him I would contact his consultant. David responded, after I had written to her, to say not to worry and that the supervisor would take care of details from here.

On mum's 80th birthday—January 10th David wrote back overnight to say that mum and dad had agreed to participate, and he would contact Tim. So, from his scant details, it seemed that they would be doing a genetic test of some sort for the immediate family. Paul was in Africa and there was no MacTel center there. They were not interested in Uncle Ernie. So, perhaps mum and dad were the key members, besides David and myself. A family effort to help figure out the mystery of our disease was an interesting, welcome, and fresh turn in the story. Later that morning, after a brutally cold walk in the park, I called to wish mum a happy birthday, and then talked to dad. He said David had been in touch about it, but that he was vague. He went to on say that they were interested in looking at their (mum and dad's) retinas, which was a surprise to me. I told him I figured they were going to do a simple blood test, and did not know any more details either. Perhaps David did not know what would be involved at this point. Dad said, again, that his information was "vague" and went on to say that he had had so many blood tests in recent years that there should be some floating around that they can use. I think he was only half joking, but I knew that this is not how they do research. He was starting to sound like he was worried about what was in store, given the seemingly constant and endless treatments he had been in of late. Perhaps this was one too many procedures for him. I hoped not. Then he said, "Well, if it sounds too much, I can always refuse."

I was taken aback for a moment, but then quickly understood, and agreed with him-albeit unenthusiastically. He did not want to see a doctor or a hospital unless he had to. I could understand that. I could have completed my life happily without ever taking another eye test involving letters projected onto a wall that always seemed, cruelly, just too far away. His treatments were far more intrusive and difficult than mine. But his reaction was pricking a small hole in the collaborative family mystery tour I had in my mind, and was excited about, since David contacted me about the possible MacTel Project involvement. He had messaged that mum and dad were "Happy to be involved." Now, after talking on the phone, I was not so sure. Although I thought they would participate in the end, unless it involved something arduous like travelling to Moorfield's in London, or going through retina tests. I assured dad that it was probably just a genetic test done from a small blood sample, but I also sensed that if more clarity was not forthcoming soon that some resistance to participating might start to set in. I knew I would just have to wait and see what it all involved.

The specialist whom I emailed had not responded yet, perhaps she would not, after all Moorfield's was a prestigious hospital. I was a little anxious for this storyline to progress. David did not seem to know much at this point either. I was sure information would be forthcoming on what to do next, and I left it all alone for a few days. I messaged David to say that I would wait for further details as they emerged.

I spent some time, one day, cleaning my desk area at home just before the semester began. I went through my collection of rocks which I kept in that part of my study. I kept coming back to the petrified woods that I always liked, and I set myself a goal to try cutting some of it this year. Perhaps I could cut a series of smaller stones to make a necklace for Hema? I also bought some vintage Indian wood printing blocks online, and began experimenting with printing designs and imagining painting-in the tiny flowers and foliage in some of the designs. I would need my magnifying glass, and a very thin brush but, perhaps, I could still produce something aesthetically pleasing, even if I was not cutting stones. Perhaps I could even make something that could be framed for the house, or for gifts.

On Sunday 11th I received a warm if brief email from Dr. Cathy Egan from Moorfield's Hospital. She thanked me for contacting them, and let me know that a blood sample for the MacTel project would be "fabulously useful." From here, her administrative assistant would contact LMRI in La Jolla to set things up from there in terms of the best MacTel site for me to visit to give a sample. She also told me that they were interested in non-affected family members, in order to explore early detection—so Tim and Paul would be useful for this, but probably only Tim would be able to participate. From her email it sounded like they were assuming we would travel to a MacTel research site to give a blood sample. The nearest for me would be at Bascom Palmer Eye Center in Miami. La Jolla, although a beautiful place to visit, would be a long and expensive trip just to provide a blood sample. Would mum and dad have to go to London to do the same? I doubted that they would, as that would be an arduous journey for them. But we would all have to wait to hear from them for the next step, and for each of us to figure out how we would be involved.

A few days later, David messaged briefly to explain that he would need to have his appointment first and, when confirmed that it is indeed MacTel by someone from the research team, they would then set me up for an appointment in Miami. We had spent most of our lives, particularly after the age of 16 or so, trying so hard to be separate—to be different and apart from each other. We consciously chose different subjects to study in high school. I still remember the moment when he asked me to make sure we were not in any of the same classes in high school. I agreed, it was time then to shake off the "twin" label we both found so annoying and confining. We chose different colleges to go to in different cities, and even ended up in different countries after graduating, perhaps partly at least due to this instinct to separate—to be individuals, finally. No one knew we were twins unless we told them, or unless it was a very rare occasion when we were in the same place and time. Yet it did strike me as slightly ironic that, here we were all these years later, experiencing being twins again, albeit mostly on the level of a genetic connection through a common health struggle. We had the same chronic disease, reminding us that we had the same genes, and now our narrative journeys were converging once again as we aged into this unfolding condition. The truth was that it would be helpful for us to collaborate moving forward if we were to understand the genetics of what we had individually, and whatever knowledge came with that in terms of its cause and likely path forward. Whether the process would bring us closer as twins or as a family, or if it would just be *useful* for our own personal narratives of what was happening to us, was yet to be discovered.

On January 16th, the day before Hema's birthday, I gave her a birthday card I had printed from one of my Indian wood print blocks. I had painted in the details with a very fine tipped paint brush, with the help of a magnifying glass that had a small light in it. It was a green vine of two interweaving strands. I gave them yellow flowers and raspberry fruits where the print block had outlined these things. She seemed to really like it—saying she would frame it. I told her to wait until I produced a really perfect one. She joked that she saw me working on it, and wondered what it was for. She probably guessed that it was for her birthday. She took a picture of it so that she could send it to her sisters. Perhaps I had found a new form of creative expression.

Solo Time

In early February Hema, quite suddenly, got a hankering to go back to India to visit her sisters and parents. Part of it was that it was an opportune time—she was free and could go for an extended trip of five weeks, and fares were lower in this off season period. Part of it was to join in the celebration of her uncle's 60th birthday—an event of high significance. But a major part was just to spend time with her sisters and parents whom she had not spent time with in many years. So, I would be solo for five weeks for the first time since we had been together. When it came time to leave, she was more nervous than I was. The day she left she wept, and told me that she would never forgive herself if anything bad happened to me while she was gone. She was worried about me. I assured her that I would not be driving anywhere unusual, and that the days were getting longer, which meant better light at the beginning and end of the days. I thought I would be fine, although I was silently also a little worried. Hema had become the person who organized things that needed doing for the house, bought groceries, and did most of our driving. She was the center of my life now in every way. I knew I would miss her as much as she would miss me, and I cried with her on the day she left.

As it came time to drop her at the airport I worried, again silently, a little about making the correct turn on my way home alone. The roads around the airport had been reconfigured recently, and the signs were often placed right where the decision to turn should have already been made. I was fine, it turned out that there was a sign indicating the turn well before the final sign at the actual exit turn. But the small details that I had not had to worry about for a while played on my mind. In transit to Newark, and while boarding, she texted constantly, missing me. The last text was a selfie of herself sitting in her seat where she would be until Frankfurt. The caption "Love you" would be her last words for a while.

That evening, as I checked my email accounts, the all too familiar "no connection" popped up again. DAMN! This would be the fifth time in two weeks that we had called for technical help from AT&T as our wireless signal failed yet again. We were convinced last time they had fixed it—it was showing five nice solid green bars when Chad, the technician, left. Now it was back to its flickering, fleeting, two or three bars. As I fell asleep, the knowledge that, if she emailed or messaged me overnight in transit through Germany and on to India, I would not get it the next morning. The forced silence between us was painful and suddenly it felt like a very big world. The next morning I had a full day of work planned but my internet connection was down, and I could not go to the office because we had plumbers arranged here for the day. I was stuck, irritated, and sad. This, and the fact I could not get a message to or from Hema, made this a terrible start to this solo time.

Around 9 am I got a call back from Chad saying he had a modem for me, but I would have to meet him somewhere to get it as he had another job to do. I could not quite place the location he mentioned, but I would call him back later to rendezvous on it. He sounded reluctant to come all the way over to our house to drop it off. I immediately worried about trying to find an unfamiliar street in traffic. On the very first day she was gone I would have to drive somewhere unfamiliar, which was the very thing I told Hema I would not do while she was gone. Hema would be able to get us there without a problem! Just after this call, James the plumber arrived with the bad news that, as they were short-handed, he would not get everything done in a day. Again, more chaos than I was used to handling alone. This was definitely a challenging first day alone for me.

The modem was up and down again, and obviously needed changing, so I called chad again the next morning. He was working in Adams farm-a nightmare of a place to find anyone for me. It is a huge neighborhood where everything looks the same. He gave me the option of coming to pick up or wait until the afternoon when he might be over this way closer to our house. I gambled on the latter. Somehow during the day he arranged for a fellow technician to meet me at his job site just around the corner on Primrose and pick up a brand new modem. I googled it, found the guy, and came home and installed it, all by myself! I was thrilled to have reliable wireless again. Hema could Skype from Chennai tomorrow, and I could finish the book chapter I was working on from home. I settled down a bit. Wireless was fixed if only for a few days, and by late Saturday afternoon 7th February the plumbing was also just about finished.

I settled in quite well, sticking to familiar routes and routines while Hema was gone. She had told me that several people would invite me over for dinner while she was gone. I was reluctant to do this, and I think she let people know that I probably would not be driving alone to their houses at night. One by one people checked in, just asking me how I was doing but not really extending any invitations for me to come over. Hema cautioned me to be careful of how I refused invitations from Indians, and I kept this in mind, but did not really need to for a while.

I received a postcard from the DMV reminding me that my license renewal was coming up in July, and that I could set an appointment earlier if I wanted to. Part of me wanted to get in and get it over with. However, I knew that it might be a difficult turning point, and set this aside as I had five months still on my current license. But this did bring up some momentary fears about not being able to drive.

The day before Valentine's Day, I received a bright and friendly call from Jennifer in San Diego. She was the link person I had been given to contact by the folks at Moorfield's Hospital, once David had been registered in the MacTel project. She would eventually link me with a person in Miami who would coordinate me coming down there for tests, and to give a blood sample. If diagnosed with MacTel, they would discuss the possibility of me enrolling in the upcoming clinical trial which she mentioned. After some preliminary questions confirming that I had been diagnosed with MacTel, and my location in the US, the most memorable moment of the conversation occurred as follows:

Jennifer:	"Are you an *identical* twin?"
Me:	"Yes, identical."
	Pause.
Jennifer:	"I hope this doesn't sound bad, but we *really* want your blood!"
	Both laugh.
Me:	"I can imagine! And I am glad to give it. We must be quite the jackpot for genetic research!"

We both laughed again, and I thought to myself that something good may come of being a twin after all.

She went on to explain the process of collecting blood, and where it would be sent for analysis; tests they would do and where they would be sent for interpretation; and the paperwork needed to enroll me in the MacTel project. I would need to visit Miami within the next two months to have a possibility of participating in the experimental study, which would involve another trip back to Miami to have an implant placed into one eye. The implant could be a placebo or the medication they were testing. I did not follow all of the details, as I was more focused on the time frame. Hema was out of town, and I was in the midst of a very busy spring semester. I explained to her that I would need Hema to go with me. I could not imagine having a day of eye tests, and being dilated, only to find my own way back to a hotel somewhere in Miami. I could do it, but I very much did not want to. On the phone the next day, Hema offered to go as soon as she returned, but I thought she would need some time at home before another trip. It was all to be worked out, but it was great to have some progress evolving. I wanted to let David know what was happening but the wireless connection was out again and, by now, Chad was not responding to my texts for help!

The Sunday right after Valentine's Day, John and his old friend Jim would meet me at the movie theatre across town at the old mall to see The Kingsman—a silly British action/spy movie. It would be the furthest I had ventured out alone, particularly at night, in a long time. I was nervous. I needed gas so I went to the gas station, then doubled back to head towards the mall on a familiar route. It was a little added driving, but this way I could visualize the turns and that helped me relax. On the way there I hoped no one would get behind me impatiently and make me nervous. Luckily the movie place, which I had never been to before, was right where I visualized it, and all went well. I missed Hema, not just because she would have driven, but it just seemed so odd going out to a movie without her. On the way back home afterwards I debated—turn right and go over by campus and the familiar but longer way home. Or, take the slight risk to turn left across High point road and come back over Holden. I pulled up to the light and decided to go left. I hoped for a green arrow to go left so that I would not have to coordinate with oncoming traffic. But I was not sure if I would know if it was an arrow or a solid light. Luckily someone pulled up in the turn lane next to me and, when it turned green, they set off, so I knew it was an arrow. All went well.

Tuesday, two days later, we were snowed out of campus. No classes all day. Hema called to chat and to see if I had talked with the link person in Miami yet. I had not, but I assured her I would soon, I smiled to myself—Hema was staying on the story even from Bangalore, and even after an all-night bus ride from Chennai the night before!

I contacted Cristy in Miami, and messaged David to let him know I was making arrangements to be tested and enrolled, and to provide a blood sample. I also mentioned to him the implant trial study that they might enroll me for. He responded within a couple of days to let me know that he was not eligible for the implant study, but he would be part of the genetic research. I imagined the same would be true for me, and I just waited for the word from Miami.

When I called during the time Cristy was available, I misread a seven for a one in her number and ended up getting through to another office. The woman was helpful but when I told her I was trying to find Cristy Rodriguez, she told me, "Sir, we have several Cristy Rodriguez's!" I started over and, realizing my misread, called the correct number and left her a message. She returned my call the following Monday and directed me to call another person to register all of my details before calling her back and making an appointment with her. I agree to do this, but could not help thinking to myself that getting there to give them my blood was starting to feel like a slow and cumbersome process. I delayed for several weeks on taking this next step, until Hema was back home in March.

Relational Time

When Hema returned, I was waiting at the point closest to where passengers come out into the general area. I waited in one of the rocking chairs until she texted to say that she was waiting for her carry-on bag, and that she would be out in a few minutes. As I hugged her, she was more concerned that, while she was walking towards me, she was waiving to me without me returning her wave. Was I as excited to see her as she was me? She had to add a little drama to the personal and intimate moment happening in public, which was always an uncomfortable context for her. I told her that I waived as soon as I could make out it was her. Did she want me to waive at people not knowing it was her for certain?! We laughed. It was so good to see her again, and have her back home.

That weekend I called home and had her talk to my mum and dad, who were also very happy to talk to her, and to know that she was back home. As she handed the phone back to me, and I went through the ritual topics and questions of our weekly call, I asked if they had heard from David. Mum, who has always gravitated to the grimmer side of description, added: "They've taken his license off him!"

"What, really? He can't drive anymore?" I questioned.

"Yes, he's finished now." She added (meaning that his driving days were finished, not that he was finished).

I could not believe it. Did the driving authorities there have a direct link to the medical people, I wondered. How would they know he was having problems? Did he tell them? As I was talking to mum and reacting with shock on the phone, Hema was mouthing, "What happened?" so I signaled to wait a minute. As I hung up she wanted to know what had happened, so I told her that David's license has been taken away from him.

"Why" she asked?

"Because he can't see!" I replied, very curtly, as if she should have known, given that he has the same disease as me. I found myself momentarily annoyed that she did not immediately understand. After all, this might be my story soon too.

I messaged David to ask him for details. He wrote back soon to explain: "Folks mentioned your driver's license, what's happened with that? I opened."

"Only that the consultants have said that I should not drive-so I don't drive now-real pain." He replied.

"Oh, Ok. Yes that's really tough. I am not far away."

"Have you got an appointment booked in Miami yet?" He shifted to requesting an update on the enrollment in the genetic study.

Hema and I were concerned, but talked instead about the fact that his wife could drive, and that he took the train to work. They lived in a village so he could get by with walking. Driving was not as much of a necessity there, for him, as it was here, for me. I also thought to myself, but did not voice it to Hema, that things were declining alarmingly quickly for him. To stop driving is a major turning point in this journey, and he must be going through some difficult emotions around it. Our message conversation above, obviously, included no such discussion of experience or emotions between us other than for him to describe it as a pain—an inconvenience, and for me to briefly acknowledge that it must be tough. Even while acknowledging that it must be a tough time, I quickly related his experience to myself by adding that I am not far away. Was I empathizing, or simply turning the conversational moment to be about me? It is ambiguous. Perhaps it was some of both. How would he read the conversation, I wondered to myself? Here we were again, pushing away from our commonality, sticking to the facts, while being never very far from a misunderstanding.

Hema and I found a bit of humor in the difference between his and mum's version of the event. Did she really have to make it sound like someone almost grabbed his license from his hands?! We laughed to get away from the darkness of his news, as his news was sad for him, and portentous for me. We could not help thinking that this semantic gap was quite typical of how Mum would relay almost any story to us—erring toward a grayer, more pessimistic, description.

· 17 ·

GETTING TO THE END OF A GOOD YEAR—GETTING TO MIAMI

Over spring break I caught up on a huge amount of grading, as well as some marathon viewing of the world cup cricket tournament from Australia and New Zealand. My eyes could feel the strain. The deep fatigue from staring at screens had seeped from my eyes throughout the front of my brain and I had to just rest for a day or two before school started up again.

In my annual review report I explained how "my career goals and my encroaching visual impairment have made me very selective of how I spend my time" I was trying to explain clearly that I did not want to sign up for committees around campus in which I had no interest. To me my time was precious, and I was not going to waste it trying to look busy for the sake of a good "service" review. The review did not address this point. Still I thought it was worth stating my position clearly and in writing. From now on I would not be saying yes to everything but, rather, would be focusing more on what I wanted to do, and to achieve.

I had slipped on the task of making the call to organize the trip to the eye institute in Miami. I was just bogged down in working on the new books, and the big push to the end of the semester. Hema began pushing me to make the call at the end of March on the off chance that we might combine the trip with something for our anniversary in May. I was a little skeptical of the celebratory frame given the battery of exhausting tests I would be going through, and the early onset of the bright and hot spring in Miami, but this was starting to emerge as a sort of combo plan.

A week after the phone conversation about David's driver's license with mum and dad, they clarified more of the story. Apparently he had gone to get his license renewed. He had to check or not check a box that disclosed something about having any eye conditions. Because he checked the box, he had to go for a follow up test to "read license plates, and what have you" as dad put it. A few days later he received a letter denying his license renewal. I felt for him as I imagined the existential moments when he checked the disclosure box, and when the letter of denial arrived through his letter box. Although he was only a walk from his train station, and his wife could drive them when needed, I realized it was a major and difficult moment for him. I also wondered why he had not filled me in on this part of the story. Perhaps this all happened since he told me his doctors had advised him to stop driving. And yet I had not received any follow up details from him. There was always a chance that it was not accurate also, given the discrepancy from the story I got from my parents a week before. Nevertheless, shortly after this information, Hema picked up the topic in a conversation with me. She emphasized that she would go with me for the renewal process, and that she would also renew hers when I did. She would be there in case I failed, although at the end of March, and still a few months away from the deadline, we did not explicitly frame it like this.

I am not sure why, but I became a worse back seat driver. Easter Sunday we went to the Indian store for some things, and I oohed and ahhed worriedly if she drifted in the lane or turned a corner too close to the curb. Later, as we left the parking lot at Bed Bath and Beyond, I was complaining about other drivers also. She pulled over and told me I could drive if I wanted to! It was so bright I did not want to, so I quietened down on the constant critical comments. Far more stressful than the last part of the semester was the upcoming driving test—looming closer all the time. As we drove along there were moments when I imagined not being allowed to drive anymore, and I am sure this anxiety was somehow at the root of my bad passenger behavior.

I know I was nervous about leaving for Austin and the conflict conference alone. It was just too expensive for her to come and it was an all-day conference over two days, so she would have been alone most of the time anyway. I was sure I would be ok, but I did not like travelling alone any more.

I had recently gotten into Indian wood block printing. I loved the vivid patterns—lotus flowers and mandalas, elephants and mangos (paisley) and other Indian inspired shapes. I used a lot of paper practicing, but I told myself that as long as I could see, I was going to create—to express myself creatively somehow. I made prints with particular people in mind and, Easter Sunday I posted the first two that I was comfortable for people to see to Fb. They were simple patterns, but the vivid red lotus on white paper made for clean and striking images. Perhaps this would take over as a creative outlet for a while from the rock cutting which was a bit more difficult and demanding of close vision. Later that day I had a request for a print from Mike, an old friend who had just moved into a new house. I would be glad to make one for him, and began planning a slightly bigger design as a housewarming gift for him. I also reserved the first successful print for Suresh who was visiting from DC while I would be in Austin. It was something for his bachelor pad in the U.S., where he stayed for half of the year.

At Easter, the end of the semester was beginning to come into focus. I had to cover one more topic in each class then it was all projects and presentations, and grading, from there. I still had a massive amount of work to do on research projects, but I was feeling good about the year, and May would bring some breathing room to focus on writing.

In mid-April I went to Austin for the second of their annual Conflict Conference event. I was really looking forward to it, although I really wished Hema was going with me. At the airport, she checked me in through the self-check in, which was always a little stressful for me alone. I did not want to get confused and stressed and hold the line up. I knew I would be alone coming back so I enjoyed her help in Greensboro. The words "seats assigned at gate" added to the stress. Did I have a seat or not? Why could they not tell me what my seat was when I checked in? As I passed through security, my magnifying glass alerted my bag for a closer check as it usually did. The security agent explained that it looked unusual or that it could be a weapon from the scan but, when he saw it, he was more curious about why I needed it than whether it was a weapon or not. I explained I needed it for close up reading and, carefully switching the little light on it back off, he was kind enough to wish me well on my journey, and with my eyes. On the flights coming back I took the magnifier out of my bag so it would be easier for them to see and, thus, avoided the hassle of more bag searches.

The gate assignment from Atlanta to Austin was also missing from the ticket so, in Atlanta, I also had to find the gate on the monitor. This turned out to be so far above my head it was difficult to see any of the information. Here I was again, standing closer than anyone around me and straining to see information that should have been much more easily accessible. As I waited for my plane a blind woman with a white stick came briskly by, and made it all look so easy. How had she mastered the information hurdles, I wondered?

I had chosen the same hotel, mainly because I did not want to struggle to find directions from somewhere different. I also wanted to create a bit of continuity for the conference last year. I was hoping to make this trip an annual tradition as it meant a lot to me to be here among esteemed and like-minded colleagues. Things went well at the hotel, although I remember having to lean in very closely to see the items names on the breakfast buffet lids. No one seemed to mind, although I was a little self-conscious at leaning in so close to food, albeit covered.

The first day of the conference included my morning presentation. As I greeted the audience I explained that I was visually impaired and that it was difficult for me to have bright lights shining in my eyes—so I had not created a power point presentation. I proceeded to circulate my handout and pressed on despite feeling very out of date in my presentational media of choice. More than the lights, which may not have been directly in my eyes, was the issue of the slide changer. Small control gadgets like this, which could be quite varied in design were stressful to deal with, especially in front of an audience. Everything went well. Although by mid-afternoon I felt the deep ache of eye fatigue setting in as I had squinted at numerous presenters and their power point slides for hours by then. In the late afternoon a Spanish colleague who sat behind me again this year asked if a group of us seated around him was up for some live music after the conference. We would be in the conference until around 6 pm. I did not want to say no, but privately I was dreading the idea as, by now, my eyes and head were deep into the pain of fatigue. I wanted to get back to the hotel and take some Advil and go to sleep, but I also did not want to seem like a bore. It was awkward, but as the last round of presentations wrapped up, I carefully packed things into my bag ready for a quick clean exit. As the session ended I got up with my things and turned around to explain that I was tired and was heading back to the hotel. He guessed from my bag in hand non-verbal behavior that this would be the story.

"Oh you're not staying for the round table discussion?" He asked, politely avoiding the more personal issue of skipping dinner with them.

"No, I am really tired and am heading back." I replied and just kept moving. He and the small group looked disappointed but I pressed on, looking forward to the walk home and some quiet solitude with my eyes closed. I walked back to my hotel with Phil Glenn and we chatted and caught up on news. He was meeting his wife at their hotel several blocks past mine. It was a pleasant late spring afternoon in Austin as we strolled past the beautiful live oaks and tame pigeons of south campus. I was glad to get outside and have the hotel up ahead, and he was glad to have the terrible Boston winter of this year behind him. The next day I made an effort to ask how their evening out had gone, and to chat with my colleague about football and other things besides conflict to make sure my slipping away the evening before was not taken personally.

When I got back from Austin, Hema began pushing me to follow up on the calls to get to Miami and register with the MacTel project. I was stalling, looking at the more immediate grading and writing mountain that lay just ahead for me. She was right, I needed to get moving on this, and she was also trying to combine a trip to Miami with our anniversary—aware of the opportunity to make the most of the trip on the small budget we were on at the time.

On April 26th David popped up again on Facebook Messenger: "Have you been for your MacTel test yet?"

"We will go after academic year is done. This summer. I got to my specialist on Monday for 6 month follow up. Are you journaling your experience at all? I am writing a detailed account of it all. It helps." I replied.

He did not reply. I assumed he was not keeping a journal and/or had no interest in discussing why it was helpful. He may have been annoyed that I had not been yet, I did not know. A week or so later I commented that the Molton Brown candle he gave us the last time we were home was really great, to which he did reply that, yes, they are really high quality candles.

Six Month Check-Up

The drive to my six month check-up was a disaster for us. The evening before, Hema had googled the directions and had us exiting at a particular exit on I-40—182, I think it was. I had reread the appointment information, and had focused mainly on making surer we left on time to get there on time. It did not occur to me that the appointment would be at a different location from the one we had been to before, and neither of us confirmed this fact ahead of time. Nearing Winston we got confused, and both of us became stressed and me angry, which added to Hema's stress. I just wanted to get there on time. Yet Hema was convinced, rightly, that we were at a different location further along I-40W. A small note on the appointment information alerting us to the location change would have been very useful, but there was nothing. Their website had no map to the location and, as I fumbled with the phone to try to locate their number, I realized as I listened to the 8 or 9 options, there were none that matched our needs for clarity on where we were going. We called Nand who goes to the same Doctor. He guided us to the main location of the eye center in Winston and, when we got there, were told that on Monday's Dr. John is at their other location in Davie County. Bermuda Run. I felt so confused and foolish, dragging us to the wrong place. The nurse helped us get clear directions, and gave us a parking pass to get out of here free, and we were off again.

While chatting with Dr. John before the examination, I made sure to accept the blame for going to the wrong location as Hema sat with us. It was the very least I could do after causing so much stress and sucking away another half-day of Hema's life on my needs.

When Dr. John examined my new retinal images he was pleased to inform me that there was no further degeneration evident from the pictures. My retinas appeared to be stable—as stable as they would be anyway. As he showed me the image of my right eye, I asked him for clarity on how close the largest damaged spot I could see close to my fovea actually was from the fovea.

"If this was half a millimeter to the right, you wouldn't be able to see anything from this eye." He clarified starkly. One half of one millimeter and I would have been blind already in my right eye. Later, as we quietly trekked back to Greensboro, this truth swept through my head, in and out and round and round. How lucky I was that it had not blinded me. How unlucky I was to have this disease at all. And again, how lucky I was. Both at the same time.

Hema was worn out from the stress of the drama of the day and did not sleep well that night. Again I would need to get better at making sure we had directions, and that her job of driving was as low stress as possible. But, I know, I had said the very same thing before, and here we were again!

Small and Big Moments That Make a Good Year

There were always small moments of awkwardness that I experienced around campus. Just before the end of class on the second to last week of classes (April 16th) I had just handed out the codes for the students to do online course evaluations. They just got settled in to writing them when the fire alarm went off. I was disappointed as it was a great class, and I knew few of them would follow up on completing the reviews once out of the class and onto the rest of their busy days. As I stood out in the cool cloudy mid-day, a woman was waving to me from further down the pathway that leads to Ferguson building. She was, perhaps, fifty feet or so away. I waved tentatively as I did not know who she was. I was conscious that I was waving less enthusiastically than she did. It would have been easier to match her wave with enthusiasm in kind, but it was hard to wave enthusiastically at someone whom you do not recognize. It would have felt fake, like I was over-acting. She could even have been waving at someone behind me, and then I would have looked foolish. I could see dark hair and a friendly energy in the wave, but I had no idea who it was. She was also saying "Hi there" as she got closer as if I knew her well. I still had no idea who it was from her voice. As she got much closer, just a few feet away, I realized it was Jenni—one of my colleagues whom I rarely saw except for at departmental meetings. We greeted and she immediately said:

"Well I guess I *do* look different!" perhaps referring to her hair color change. She was aware that I did not recognize her.

"No," I said, "I can't see very well." I clarified, though I do not think my attempt to convey that it was not her, but that it was me, was working.

"Oh OK!" she responded with a friendly chuckle, but I think she thought it was the hair color change that was throwing me off. She changed her hair color regularly. At least she did not think I was being standoffish, which would have been an unfortunate misunderstanding. We quickly segued into talk of student evaluations, and joked about someone pulling the alarm who did not want to do a presentation or test. Others quickly joined us, and we joked about going back in the building to rescue our lunches, fire or no fire.

There were also always small moments of friction and misunderstanding. At the end of April, I was leaving for a hair-cut. The salon was all the way at the end of Horse Pen Creek Road. Hema asked me why I was leaving so early. I replied that it took a good twenty minutes to get there. She quickly realized I was going the long way round. To cut across New Garden Road would have meant I was right at the correct end of Horse Pen Creek Road without going all the way up Battleground Avenue. She told me she could not understand why I went that way. It was a good ten minutes more. For me it was a route I was familiar with, and which I could visualize. There were no left turns across traffic without an arrow, and I also quite enjoyed the long winding road. She insisted I go the other way and, again, pressed me on why I went the long way round. It just did not make sense to her. I told her that I live in a little different world from her and cannot read signs on unfamiliar routes so well. She relented and clarified where I turn. I followed her idea although, momentarily, I thought about going my old way. It cut the travel time significantly, and was an easy route.

On May 19th I finally made the call to Bascom Palmer to register and received a registration number. I emailed Cristy and told her I was ready to set up a visit to Miami this summer. I also messaged David and added a question about whether they would also still want to test Mum and Dad and Tim. He responded overnight—early morning for him, with the statement that he had tried several times to get them moving forward on the tests for the family but that they were slow. Perhaps, he thought, when my results were confirmed then they might move more quickly on their tests. Clearly he was trying to move the process along on his end. Eventually we set a tentative day to come to Maim on June 18th.

Nagging at me in June was the upcoming driving test that I was dreading. I needed to get it done before my birthday on July 4th. I began to imagine passing it with excitement and failing it with dread. If I passed it I would have some freedom and would not be a burden to Hema. If I failed it the story would be the opposite. If I did not fail it but did badly on it, would they at least let me drive locally? The thought of not being able to drive to the park for an early morning walk, and to pop in to the Fresh Market for something we needed, were sad thoughts. More significantly if I could not drive to work, and Hema got a full-time job, I would have to get cabs to and from the office. Ugh! I thought to myself. What kind of life would that be?

Sunday morning I relished an early morning drive to the park, and a walk through the woods. About half way round, my mind slipped to the thought of perhaps not being able to drive anymore and I found myself verbalizing "Oh No!" into the air several times. The heaviness of the impending moment was taking form for me. I tried to be in the moment—to shake it off amidst the slow fresh coolness of the Sunday morning, but it was not easy. I picked up some half and half on the way back at the Fresh Market, which Hema insisted on for her morning coffee. Such small moments of freedom in the woods, and small opportunities for relational thoughtfulness, seemed to depend on me being able to drive.

On Monday June 8th I got a response from Cristy in Miam stating that my appointment was set for Thursday 18th starting at 9 am. I had no indication of exactly where and no clarity on travel arrangements or where to stay. I asked if I would be needed just for the Thursday and what we do about travel and accommodation. She responded only addressing the fact that I would be needed only for Thursday. Hema and I agreed that if costs were not covered, then we would not go. Why would she not even address those questions or, if she did not know, simply state that she would look into those and get back to me? This had been somewhat of my first impression of Bascom Palmer, slow and incomplete information, and not very proactively helpful. The truth was that they were very, very busy, and I would grow to like them all very much after we visited. Hema offered to step in and manage things but I held her off for now, hoping that clarity would come.

I messaged David to tell him that I had an appointment next week, but that it had been difficult to get needed information such as whether or not they were covering expenses. He messaged back that same day saying that he had all but given up trying to follow up with the equivalent people where he was. We were having a similar experience of luke-warm responsiveness. I replied by stating that I do not think this research project (and by association the study of our disease) is what pays the bills for anyone. It is understandable that it is a second area of research interest, and everyone is busy, but it was still frustrating to have to keep nagging for clarity and information about the appointment process.

The appointment details were clarified on Wednesday morning and, given the choice between their travel agent and doing it ourselves, Hema got on the laptop and worked out the flights and accommodations in an hour. Going back and forth with their agent would have been unnecessary stress. We would stay an extra day so that she could see Miami—a place she had never been to before. I messaged David that all worked out and he messaged back overnight with a simple, "That's good." We were all set.

I thought about posting something to social media. Perhaps, making some sort of announcement about becoming a human subject for the study of the disease I have. But I did not know what to write. A personal announcement of a disease just is not appropriate on Facebook. How would people respond? What would they think? Why would I want to make any announcements at all, I also wondered? Perhaps I would work it into a comment about escaping the heat of Greensboro for Miami! Unusually, it was hotter here than down there at the moment. In the end, I thought it just too awkward and personal for Facebook or other social media. When in Miami I did a check-in from Bascom Palmer, with no additional comments on Facebook, and received a few concerned comments, most quickly from my aunt Elizabeth who had worked at an eye hospital in the UK, and from a couple of friends. I added a comment that I was donating my defective genes to the MacTel project and a couple of people wrote that they were glad I was ok and not in serious trouble.

On our first evening there, we decided to go for a walk around the area. Mostly I wanted to see where we would be going the next morning, but also we just wanted to see what was around us. We quickly realized that this was not an area for strolling and sightseeing. It was clearly an area where the medical staff worked and then left after work, and lived somewhere else. It was desolate except for a few homeless people, and not a place to look like tourists—taking pictures next to palm trees, or debating directions while looking at a map. I joked the next day about this image with one of the technicians, and he laughed, emphasizing that NO! This was not the area to do something like that. We saw the Bascom Palmer building, an efficiently designed concrete structure with a "#1 in Eye Care" banner posted on it, and we then turned around and quickly headed back to the hotel.

The next morning we checked in at the hospital after a long sweaty and circuitous shuttle ride to the clinic. It would have been much better just to walk the three blocks to Bascom Palmer. The day began with us checking in and meeting Cristy, who walked us through the upcoming day's activities. She told me I was #124 in the study, and that there was one other twin pair so far. I told her how it would be great to connect with them, but the confidentiality requirements precluded such contact. The day consisted of all of the tests I had done over the past few years multiplied by two or three, and an all-important blood sample, followed by a meeting with Dr. Rosenfeld. At each station, technicians were clearly concerned with making sure each image or test was done to his liking, and I quickly absorbed their pervasive image of him as a brilliant perfectionist. Everything had to be done according to the research protocols also. At one station the machine they wanted to use was taken up with another patient, and apparently would be for a while. There was much discussion and double checking to see if they could use an equivalent but different machine for the test. Any variability was being strictly controlled, even down to using the same machines. I quickly realized why they did not let me just drop off a genetic sample with my ophthalmologist back home!

It was freezing in the clinic, so I asked Cristy if she could find a blanket for Hema, who was patiently staying with me throughout the various stages of tests and data collection. She did, but Hema refused the blanket, stating that there were many people older than herself in the waiting rooms without blankets. The staff were friendly, helpful and playful despite their obvious caution in working for Dr. Rosenfeld. When I explained how, in Indian culture, people often politely refuse things three times before accepting, one technician asked if Hema refused my marriage proposal three times before accepting! We acted out the scene playfully, sharing a much needed laugh. When my vein would not produce any blood I joked that I lost more blood shaving with the free hotel razor that morning, and they joked back that I should have just collected that. By 1:30 in the afternoon they gave us a half hour break for lunch and then it was back to it again. Using our lunch voucher, Hema got us a quesadilla that was more than enough for two, and we sat out under the shaded courtyard with the small birds flitting around. It was a grueling day, but I was enjoying being around this team who were dedicated to the MacTel research project.

After the brief lunch break it was into the legendary imaging room where five different machines were used to take duplicate images of each retina, because Dr. Rosenfeld did not trust any one brand of machine alone! Things were building up to our meeting.

As we chatted with Crista, and Doctor Brian who met us before Dr. Rosenfeld, we found that Dr. Brian went to Duke, near us, and that he and his wife loved Asheville as much as we did. It was an enjoyable meeting, but everything was also being prepped carefully for the arrival of Dr. Rosenfeld. Were my eyes dilated enough in case he wanted to look into them? They quickly re-dilated my left eye. Was everything arranged just so? As we chatted, Crista finalized the eye donation forms, with Hema approving their use of my eyes for research upon my death. Crista wanted to know if the state of Florida could have all of my organs and we stopped short of that, and said we would think about it. I had no particular connection with Florida other than through this research that was focused on my eyes. As we chatted about things, the door behind me opened and in came Dr. Rosenfeld. We greeted and chatted briefly about our trip. He quickly switched to diagnostic questions. Where were my parents from, and were they related? Clearly he was working from a genetic framework and, perhaps the question about my parents being cousins was no less strange than the one about being a sungazer at the start of this journey. I mentioned briefly that I was writing about the experience, and he encouraged me to talk to the LMRI about my plans. He said he would like to read my research, which was very kind. He explained things carefully and precisely. When did I have injections in my eye, he asked? I could only give him approximate times. The room shuffled nervously when we did not have specific dates for him, but the discussion moved on. Hema wanted clarification on the likelihood of me passing on the disease in the event of us having a child. He assured her that there was no likely relationship in terms of passing on the disease. This was definitive clarity that she had been looking for, for a while. He examined the retinal images carefully, and explained how the bands of the retina had broken down around my fovea. I asked him if "stability" was a real state, and he quickly affirmed that it was. I asked him what he thought my long terms journey would look like, and he responded that it was impossible to predict. The valuable back and forth continued until I had no more questions, and the meeting began to come to a natural close. He waited for more questions, and when I could not think of any, I thanked him, and we wrapped up and left.

After the day's activities we walked back to the hotel and Hema went to sit downstairs as I tried to sleep for a while. I could not nap as the moments of the day were so vivid in my mind, and I went back through them over and over again. Eventually I texted her and said I could not sleep. She came back up to the room and I had tea. We showered and took a much needed break from the hotel area by taking the shuttle to Bayside Market where we walked, shopped, had some Cuban food, and listened to the live music. I bought Hema a simple cotton dress in the market that caught my eye as a thank you for being so patient with me. She wore it the next day as we toured around the city. The market was buzzing with energy which kept me going while Hema enjoyed the city vibe. On the way back to the hotel we chatted with a couple from the Bahamas who had brought their baby boy for treatment. One of his eyes had no sight, and he went through much of what I did in terms of tests that day *as a baby*. He was very cute and Hema was drawn to him, as she always was to babies. The guy asked her if we had children and she simply said, "No, no children" and the moment flattened awkwardly. There were people on the shuttle back to the hotel who had come from far and wide for treatment-often affirming the premier status of the clinic as they explained where they were from.

The next day I had set aside the whole day for whatever Hema wanted to do—touring the city by bus and boat, so that we could enjoy our time away from Greensboro a bit. My eyes were exhausted from the day before, but we needed to see Miami. We toured downtown, stopping in Little Havana for ice cream, and for Hema to buy a bag of Cuban coffee. I tried not to grumble at the heat and brightness but at times I did, which was not helpful. Getting upset over small things when we travelled was a habit of mine that irritated and stressed Hema. Then we did the beach tour which was sweltering on the London double decker bus. We did not move from the bus as it was too hot to get off, and have to wait for the next one half an hour later. We finished with a cruise around the bay to look at the city from the water, and take pictures of some of the houses on millionaire's row. It was a wonderful way to relax and be entertained visually. After this we went back to the hotel and had a cool shower and some food and drinks downstairs. I liked this little friendly hotel named "Spring Hill" which was, coincidentally, how my last name translates into its original Norse—"Spring on a hillside." As we got back up to the room, Hema asked sweetly if we could make love. I had nothing left in me except a desire to close my eyes and sleep. Instead of explaining this I got irritated, which was stupid. I know her mind was slipping back to the scene earlier that day when the Doctor explained to us that I would not pass on the disease to any children we might have.

This was the only place we had visited where Hema did not want to move, which surprised me. It was, perhaps, the sweltering bus tour and her efforts not to get sunshine on herself that made the place just too much work to really enjoy. This was a sunny, sweaty, tropical place in the summer time.

When we returned to Greensboro I checked in with David by message, to say that we were now both registered in the project, and that we had star genes! He wrote back to ask if they had confirmed MacTel, which they had, and to clarify that they had not actually taken his blood sample yet—which was probably the most important thing for them to do for the study. He had tried for months to make progress on donating a sample, but to no avail. Ironically, he could probably stop by on his lunch break to complete the task, whereas I had to make the trek to Miami. In my case, in Miami, they made sure they got everything they needed on one visit. He was frustrated, and said he had sent them his final email request before giving up on the process. I was shocked and felt bad that the team in Miami were operating on the assumption that he had donated blood before I had. I emailed Dr. Rosenfeld with this information and the next morning, in the early hours of Father's Day, he wrote back assuring me that David and my parents would be included in the study as soon as possible. I messaged David that he was going to push them into action, but I did not hear back from him. Perhaps he was waiting to see if anything changed first. That evening we watched CSI Miami, and Hema was able to identify many of the scenes and buildings we had seen there live, just days before. I did not recognize any of them.

On Friday afternoon, Hema received the excellent news that she had gotten nothing but positive reviews on the last part of her interview process with a local recruitment firm. Pending recommendations being fine, she would receive an offer soon. She would be busy again with work. I so much wanted her to find what she loved to do in life, and perhaps this was it. It would be a return to the executive search industry she had loved doing while in India years ago. If this all went through as it looked like it would, she would be able to support herself if anything happened to me, doing something that she found fulfilling, which had been a goal of mine since my vision problems began. Her happiness and security made me worry less about my eyes. I had sent a proposal to the LMRI through Jennifer and she emailed back to say that I was on the agenda for their next staff meeting to discuss my proposal. This might open up a whole now data base for me, and a line of research that would be profoundly meaningful for me. Hema and I enjoyed the rare beauty of a moment of symmetry—perhaps things were looking good for both of us at the same time.

The deadline for renewing my driver's license crept ever nearer. One Saturday evening, Hema asked me when I was planning to go, as she would go with me. She made a remark about me leaving it to the last minute and that she had to remind me. I responded, sharply, that I had left it this late because there was a good chance I would fail the eye test part of the exam. She assured me that many people with worse eyesight than mine have city restrictions, and not to worry. She encouraged me to change how I was thinking about the situation, and to think the best, so that it would come about. All of this helped, but I was still anxious. She claimed that either way it would not affect much of what we did. I explained, in concrete terms, that it would mean I could not go to the park for a walk alone. I could not run errands for us. I could not just take off to the office when I needed to. She began to appreciate my point but still asked me to expect that it would be fine, and we moved on to other things. Fueled by her recent assurance concerning the low likelihood of me passing on the disease, she wanted to revisit the idea of having a child. What could I be afraid of now that this fear was dispelled?

She wanted to take me to an "inner engineering" yoga event in DC as part of our planned trip over the 4th of July weekend, so things quickly turned to that, and what we would need to do before going. In the back of my mind it started to nag at me again that I was not making any progress on the book that was due in a month, and I started to wonder when the summer writing time had gone. We buried ourselves in cooking shows on TV that evening, and enjoyed a glass of wine that we had picked up to celebrate the fact that she had a job offer in the works. We were both excited at the prospect of her renewed career path with an executive search firm. At the same time, her new career focus pushed questions to the fore. For her, what would her demanding

YEAR 5

July 2015–July 2016

· 18 ·

SHARING EXPERIENCES

On our birthday, July 4th, I sent David a brief message to wish him a happy birthday, and to ask him if he had heard anything from the MacTel researchers in London. He replied that he had been pushing them via email, and that they said there may be a way forward in securing mum and dad's sample but that, as he put it, "They don't want a genetics sample from me just yet (they are chasing another interesting finding!)"

That's all he said, making no reference to the "happy birthday." No clarification on when they would want a sample, or specifically what else they were chasing that precluded them from taking his genetic sample. I found it bizarre, he sounded frustrated, and I think we were both disappointed, but what could I do? I was unlikely to get very far emailing the MacTel Project people again in London, and I had already emailed the contacts I had in Miami who had promised me this would move forward. They had, no doubt, moved on to other tasks as busy as they were. I did not know what had happened, and I did not know what to do next, so I just left it alone and enjoyed the Fourth of July celebrations with Hema.

On July 9th my new driver's license arrived. I was overjoyed to have this reprieve through the online renewal option now in effect in North Carolina. If I renewed it in person at the DMV, I *may* have made it through the eye test if all went well for me on the day, but this way I did not have to worry about it for eight years-*if* my eyes remained stable. I was elated. I promised the cosmos to be good, safe, and realistic in what I could do behind the wheel, and hoped this would see me through until I was 60! At fifty-three years old, this seemed a comfortably long way off. I quickly forgot all of my fear and anxiety that had been close to the front of my mind for the several months leading up to the expiration of my old license on July 4th. It struck me how much fear, stress, and even anger had been part of the past four years, and how much it had shaped my thinking and my reactions to things. Could I listen to my wife, and respond to her suggestion that I reshape my thinking in productive ways in the year ahead, so that it would not be so easy succumb to negative response patterns based on fear and, even sometimes, self-pity? Could I change enough so that I would *not* assume that her encouragement to live in the moment and not be so fearful of this disease, was a dismissal or denial of its seriousness to me? This was a deeply dysfunctional and frictional interpretive pattern of mine, as it simply ended in me denying her encouragement, at the same time that I was assuming she was denying my experience. Could I also make some important and constructive strides in my own research related to MacTel, and advocacy for MacTel patients? I wanted to pull together my experiences of the first five years with the disease as a book about these early stages, and I would make this the focus of my time ahead.

I had sent a proposal to conduct research into MacTel in conjunction with the Lowy Medical Research Institute in La Jolla shortly after my visit to Miami. They received it enthusiastically, and I was told that they would discuss the proposal at the next meeting. I did not hear anything back until weeks later when I followed up to ask how my ideas were received. As I wrote the proposal, I had imagined dedicating much of the rest of my career to the study of how people experience MacTel, and how it impacts communication and relationships. It seemed to me to be a perfect alignment of my skills and interests. Yet, it did not go very far. The response from the LMRI did include several innovations that would improve information to patients. Upgrading the information posted to the Facebook page was one that they were actively working on. I had noticed this improvement, and was glad they were reaching out in this way. I noticed only modest numbers of "likes" for the information at this point, but it was a good start, and the information was interesting and regular. One day they posted results from a recent Chinese research study that claimed a component of Licorice helped prevent neovascularization. Oddly, and probably coincidentally as it was the flavor I enjoyed, I had drunk licorice tea every day for many years. Perhaps it had made a difference?! Another time they posted the British version of the vision test for driving that included recognizing a license plate at a certain distance. I passed the online version. This was the test that my brother recently failed in person, and that lead to his permanent disqualification from driving there. The timing of this information based on our recent experiences was poignant. He was adjusting to the disruption and "pain" of not being able to drive, and I had scraped through to be able to continue driving for now.

Experimenting with forums and discussion groups for patients was another improvement that I welcomed, and would join enthusiastically if and when they became available. Sharing experiences and support with fellow Mac-Tel patients was something I missed having in the past four years. Improving the information on the LMRI web-site for patients was another great idea, and I noted to myself that I would check in occasionally to see what they had posted. These were all good signs that the information environment for patients was improving. The research proposal in which I would collect and examine narratives of patients was listed at the end as a future possibility, but not something that they wanted to pursue at this time. I was a little disappointed, but understood. I wanted to be part of the work of the Institute, even in some small way, in developing peoples' understanding of the lived experience of the disease. Perhaps I would find another way to collect narratives and conduct the research. Perhaps, as had been the case up to this point, I would focus on writing my own experiences.

Summer Weddings

Summer was, of course, wedding season, and this summer we had two to attend. One was the Pakistani wedding of my former student, Sidra, and her soon to be husband, Imran. The wedding reception was full of color and sparkle—particularly the dresses of the young women. I loved the spectacle, and found myself staring at the vivid red dresses and black dresses so full of glittery flowing life. I enjoyed and appreciated being able to see color so much (I expected to lose much of my color acuity while under my previous diagnosis of cone dystrophy). Sidra's father came over and told Hema to "watch me"!-mistaking my interest in the dresses for the young women wearing them. It was a cute moment, and it was good to see her parents enjoying the celebration so much, but it really was about the colors! Hema and I stayed close to each other. She was an Indian among Pakistani's, and neither of us knew many of the other people—as friendly as they turned out to be.

The second wedding was an Indian wedding. Also full of color, though different from the Pakistani wedding. This time we both knew many of the people from the Greensboro and Winston-Salem community of Indians. While we were milling around in the lobby area before the event began, Hema disappeared with her Indian lady friends, as she often did at gatherings. Indian gatherings tend to separate by gender, an ancient habit that persisted. I wandered around a bit as I often did when she disappeared. Just as I began to feel a little lost, I heard a voice from the side calling my name as I walked past. She was waving. I did not know who it was, so I was slow to react. She waved and called again as if to ask why I was not responding. It was Anjana. It just seemed awkward to explain that I was slow to react because I could not recognize her face. So, I simply greeted them and joined their family for a few minutes. Perhaps she just thought I was in my own little world as I wandered by, and perhaps I was. The enduring truth in this, and many other moments like it, was that it was extraordinarily difficult to explain to people that you cannot see certain things well, such as faces, when they can see the same things clearly. People tend to think that what they see is what you see, and it is not necessarily true. Perhaps someone could create an App that simulates a MacTel eye view of the world, so that people with healthy vision could look at the world through their phone camera as if they had MacTel? It would certainly help build understanding and empathy.

Back to School—Sharing Personal Experiences

With weddings and summer activities all but over, classes began for fall 2015 again in mid-August. During the first week, several students from last semester came by to say hi who were taking classes close to my office. It was an all too familiar scene for me: They typically stand in the open doorway of my office and say hi, to see if I remember them, and if it is ok to come in and visit. I wave them in, after what must seem like a long pause while I try to recognize them but often cannot from that distance. In that moment, I wonder what they are thinking … Does he remember me? Is he surprised to see me wanting to stop by and say hi …? I should ask what is happening in that pause, just to know. But I have not so far. As they walk in, I tell them that I cannot see very well and did not recognize them, but I rarely get the sense that they understand that this is what is happening. They cannot relate to what I am saying, because they always recognize me from where they are standing in the scene. When I say that I did not recognize them because I cannot see well, people usually chuckle, perhaps as if I were making an excuse for not remembering their name. I began to think about how I might bluff through these awkward moment better, calling them in warmly as if I know exactly who they are, while avoiding the need to use a specific name until I know who they are. The risk here is that I might wave someone in warmly, pretending to know them, but who are strangers simply asking when the Math help center next door to me will be open. This would be awkward and embarrassing. The center never seems to post operating hours on the door or wall, so I do get several people asking me questions just because my office is next door.

Thursday afternoon of that first week, I was meeting with a new graduate student—Maria—to talk about common interests in studying disability, and so that she could interview me for a class assignment. I was facing the doorway as we talked. A face slowly appeared from the left of the doorway and almost playfully waited for a reaction. I did not know who it was, but I knew they were relatively dark skinned and female. I also know that someone who appears like that—poking their head around the doorway—must know me well. This narrowed things, but not enough. I waved her in, even though I was in the middle of an appointment. She was my wife. I recognized her definitively just as she stepped forward, at first from her shape and size—her silhouette, and then as more interior details quickly filled in. We chatted, and I introduced her to my graduate student. Then I walked her out of the building as she has to go back to work. That evening, after a nice dinner out to celebrate the end of the first teaching week, she took me back to that moment in the office. She wanted to know if I could not recognize her from the doorway. I assured her that I could not, and joked it away saying that faces are hard for me from that distance, but much easier if I am expecting someone. I was not expecting her, as she was busy at her downtown office until late these days. Perhaps this clarified whatever she was thinking about that moment in my doorway, when I paused momentarily before responding to her. A couple of days later I was curious enough to ask her what she was thinking in that moment when I did not recognize her. Perhaps I did not act surprised when she was trying to surprise me? She simply said that she was wondering at what point I would recognize her. It must have felt like a long awkward moment for her in the doorway as it did for others.

Before I knew it, it was week six, and the equinox—Wednesday September 23rd. We would be dimming down towards the darkest day of the year for the next quarter. This would usher in the more limited driving days for me, as the nights would begin to get darker earlier, and the morning would stay darker longer. This was not my favorite quarter of the year, but we would muddle through somehow, driving when possible and otherwise staying close to home—unless Hema drove. At least my daily routines were relatively normal and stable at this time. I was driving to and from work, which freed Hema up to stay for her long days building her career in executive recruitment and placement. We were busy and productive, and things were rolling along well for both of us.

On Thursday 24th the MacTel group posted an invitation for patients to share experiences. It was a turning point in moving from sharing information on research findings—however relevant and applicable—to inviting communication with and between MacTel patients. It was great to see this development, but I was so busy with book writing and classes that I failed to participate at this time. Perhaps I could make time later to get involved in this excellent opportunity?

In early October we had about two weeks of grey gloom and rain following a major storm off the east coast. The gloom was a welcome rest for my eyes from the brightness. I could see so much better not having to fight the bright sun while driving and walking around campus. But it got to the point where I was happy to see the brightness return when it did. I was beginning to feel gloomy myself. The gloom was good for my eyes, but the brightness was good for my brain. These days, weather became more important for me as it involved a constant back and forth, and even struggle, of light and dark.

On a Wednesday after class, I met with Lana, one of my students. She was a regular visitor last semester when I had her for CST 207 Relational Communication and she had planned to come by this semester but could not until now. She confided in me about her advising experience—feeling that she was supposed to have a "path" or career direction going into that conversation but she did not. She found the advising conversation frustrating as she could not articulate a direction—hoping rather that one might emerge from the classes she was hoping to sign up for. She was caught in a conundrum—feeling like she should have a plan before the courses enabled her to create a plan. I helped her think through what courses she might instinctively find interesting, thinking that a direction might come with that. As we talked, somehow she transitioned to a more personal topic as she began to describe her childhood experiences with her own eye problems. She recalled being a nine year old, when she was asked to wear a patch on her left eye in order to strengthen her right eye. The patch had some sort of design on it that was meant to appeal to her age group, and perhaps even make it look cool, but she remembered *vividly* that it did not help. She broke her leg on vacation on the first day. With a patch and crutches she drew the obvious cruelty from schoolmates, with pirate themed name calling.

Adding more to her interesting personal story, she recalled being expected to wear glasses which had one very thick lens for her afflicted eye, and one less thick lens for the other one. She was horrified at this prospect, as this would have put her solidly in the "not cool" or nerdy school group. She was telling me her "ugly duckling" story, and I gave her story support when I told her that she had blossomed since then. She is an attractive and lively person who I had grown to like as a student, and she had grown to confide in me. I asked her the name of her disease. She knew it was a long name, and that it is a degenerative disease, but she could not remember it specifically. I could relate, as the four word name of my disease took a lot of practice for me to remember at first. Her disease left her with almost no sight in her left eye, but she assured that her right one compensated. I asked her if she drives at night and she said, not much. Somehow she passed through the eye test of the driver's exam while still failing the eye test. She was lucky. She did not know how it happened but she took the lucky break, and now drives as if she is fine. Then she confided that, since then, she has avoided going to the eye doctor for check-ups. I told her she should go regularly as I had learned to do, and that technology and treatment may have improved in the ten years since her early experiences.

"Maybe I will" she responded, though not entirely convincingly.

She asked me if I had had surgery for my eyes. I told her no, but that I had injections, as I had talked about in class, to handle swelling retinas. I told her about my trip to Miami, and my signing off on their use of my eyes upon my death. I elaborated that they would fly up to get them as they would be working against the clock. She played along with the extraordinary scene, saying that it must feel good to be so sought after, special! We laughed.

"Well, yes and no!" I responded, and she immediately got it. It is not the sort of "special" any of us would like.

She surprised me by revealing that she stopped indicating a willingness to donate organs on her license, as she had heard it meant that they would try less hard to keep you alive if you are willing to donate. I said I could not imagine that could be true but we agreed on "you never know!"

"The Hippocratic Oath is fuzzy" she said.

"Yes it could be," I agreed.

After all, as she went on to point out, there is a huge shortage of transplant organs, and "there you are" indicating that the logical conclusion not to mark oneself as a donor seemed obvious. As we chatted, a person walked by and waved to me in my office. I told Lana that I did not know who she was as I waved anyway, and we shared a humorous moment about it. She asked if I could recognize her from where she was sitting across from me and I could, and especially as I knew who she was my brain can make up the difference. We agreed that, even when you explain to people your vision limitations, it is hard for them to empathize because that's not what they see through their eyes. "People don't get it", we agreed, creating a moment of commonality despite having very different diseases.

On Thursday October 21st I got an email from Wake Forest to remind me of my appointment next week in Winston. I told Hema and she responded, quietly, that she would make arrangements to take a half day off. This meant she would lose a half day of the precious few leave days she had, and half a day's pay. I knew this time off was not what she needed, and I felt bad about it, but I had no other way of getting there and back. I was also due for my regular optometrist check-up on Friday of the same week, and received a reminder from them also. So, my eyes would be cycling back into being the focus of my attention next week, after six months of relative peace.

· 19 ·

RED DOTS, INVITATIONS, AND THE COMMUNICATION OF CARE

A Shaky Stability Narrative

On Wednesday October 28th we made the trek to Winston for my appointment with Dr. John. I went through the usual acuity test and photographic images as we normally did. On the wall of the consulting room to my right, where I waited, were framed images of diseased retinas. They had titles on the middle of the bottom part of the frames, like art, naming the diseases. They were otherworldly images, like oddly colored planets somewhere out there in vacuous space. Planets with red fiery atmospheres and grey lost continents. Planets with stories to tell—perhaps once fertile and green, and now hot or icy and dying. These were pictures of the retinas of people just like me, but with a variety of other diseases. Perhaps my pictures would be up on this hall of fame wall one day, I thought to myself.

Dr. John came in and greeted us warmly, remembering me and my wife. Hema had sat in the same chair last time, patiently and closely observing the scene before her as she did now. As we chatted, he asked me if I had experienced any changes, and I explained that I could not identify any new problems, or perceive any decline since the last time I came. I told him about our trip to Bascom Palmer in Miami, and he was pleased to hear that I had registered with the MacTel project. He questioned me about how my brother was doing, and I could not relay much, other than that he was still unable to register with the MacTel project in London. He explained that they might have enough of our demographic for the study, and may need types of relatives other than siblings. We chatted about my progress on writing about the experience. He wanted to know a little more about how communication related to this, so I gave a simple practical example of how the communication around the eye test at the beginning of the appointment may well impact how people perform on the test. He was intrigued, and asked if I could come and do a talk some time for the residents and staff. I would be happy to, I confirmed.

We shifted frames momentarily to look closely at the retina images. Just when I thought I was ok, still stable, and that we would be out of here early this time, he noticed two tiny red dots on my left eye which he assured me were not there the last time I came. Ugghhh! I felt the news like a body thud. I did not want two red dots to appear, but there they were nonetheless. I had no choice. These were signs that dreaded neovascularization in the, as yet largely unaffected, left eye was starting to happen. "Here we go again," I thought, fearfully, to myself. He brought in one of his residents to show her the images. We went through a slightly awkward moment where he introduced me as Dr. Kellett to her. I shook her hand and reintroduced myself as Pete. She introduced herself as Doctor something … more awkwardness, and we shifted quickly to focus on the red dots. He then sent me for another image to confirm what he had spotted. We would not be getting out of here early, and Hema's desire for a much needed rest when we got home before going back to work evaporated instantly. We would be here for a while longer, and I felt bad for both of us, but mostly for her. After confirming his suspicions, he explained that he would need to see me again in three months instead of six. "Ugggh!" I responded, silently, again. Another thud up against my now shaky "stability" narrative. That did not sound good at all. He assured me that I did not need an injection this time, but that we would need to keep a close eye on the changes in the left eye. It sounded ominous, but I knew it was to be expected as things progressed over the years. I knew I would need more injections at some point. I just ached with hope for this to be later rather than sooner. It struck me momentarily that, when doctors define diseases as "progressive," patients understand them as "declining", the exact opposite but, semantics aside, we were very much in this together.

After a quick lunch at our favorite Indo-Chinese restaurant in Winston-Salem, Hema's choice for having driven us, we hurried home so that Hema could drop me off and go back to work for a long afternoon of calls and meetings. As she left for a long and busy afternoon, I lay down to rest my eyes and to sleep for a while. Laying there, I felt the urgency of the two books I had currently in motion and close to finished. Editing was so sight intensive that my mind focused entirely on making constructive progress on this aspect of my life more than anything else. I wanted to say the things I needed to say while working on the regular screen of my lap top was easy. After a short sleep, I spent the afternoon getting the first draft of the manuscript of the first book finalized and ready for our editor. I wrote a note to Tom, my co-author, that it was finished. I wrote to three people I could think of to review the manuscript for the publisher. That evening I had already heard back with an affirmative from one. My instinct was to try to make progress on something tangible, and it felt good to push the book forward on a day with such a swirl of mixed results and emotions.

That night I messaged my brother David partly to respond to his comment about taking mum and dad to the pantomime at Christmas, and partly to ask how his eyes were doing. Dr. John's question about how he was doing left me stumbling for an answer, as I had no new information on his condition. I realized I had not asked anything about his eyes and vision in a while. I simply added "how are the eyes?" to the end of the Christmas discussion. He wrote back the same day—late in the evening in London to say, "Eyes are a real pain. Can't see peoples facial expressions unless up quite close. Makes everything a bit harder. Must arrange to get genetics test."

Facial recognition and the information conveyed through expressions was also a struggle for him. I could completely empathize. It did make everything harder. I responded affirming his struggle and encouraging him to try to set up his test: "Yes I understand. People stand in my office doorway and when I don't know who they are they think I have forgotten them! Will be good to get the genes donated."

I assume he understood but he did not respond. Neither did he ask me for any clarification on what was happening with my eyes.

Hema had been revisiting the idea of us having our own child. She went back and forth on it. Mostly forth. She really wanted a child. One evening she said that she was not sure she wanted to have a child, as having two babies would be difficult to handle! I asked her what she meant. She told me that she sees me struggling with small things and getting frustrated and angry easily, and that this worried her. Would a child be too much for her with me potentially dealing with more vision difficulties down the road? It was a conversation that neither one of us enjoyed. It was awkward. Too many unknowns were tangled up with too many hopes and dreams.

One day in my 11 am conflict communication class, I noticed that a student on the back row in the corner was difficult to see. I said his name and looked at him as if waiting for confirmation that it was him. He said "I am showing my face. Yes it's me" I clarified that it was not about his hoodie, or cap, both of which he was wearing, but my difficulty seeing clearly that far back in the room. I told him he was just at the edge of where I can see clearly. To my surprise he connected with me, telling me that he also cannot see well, and is close to blind in one eye. I had no idea, and appreciated him sharing his situation.

Travelling Alone

In mid-November, the National Communication Association conference was about to happen. I was presenting three papers at the conference in Las Vegas. I worried slightly about travelling alone. Signing in at the airport, trying to see flight information, and the thought of being in a huge hotel without Hema, were among the worries I kept mostly to myself. Hema told me not to be fearful. She even told me to try gambling. To *try things*. Travelling turned out to be fine. I did find the conference center hotel to be dark and cluttered in the lobby—my guess was that it was dark in order to highlight the bright and colorful gambling machines. It was cluttered with slot machines and card stations. This was Vegas, I told myself! It was strange, but I found my way around well for the most part, once I got my bearings.

Travelling back to Greensboro I was lucky to be on the same plane as my colleague Cerise. When we got to the airport, she helped me with the process of paying for the cab using my debit card, which can be awkward, as cabbies are usually in a hurry to leave, and the screen on their device is small. She also helped me while checking in to get the baggage tags and boarding passes. We decided to get some lunch before the flight as it was a long day's journey back. Gladly, she helped me read the menu that was posted up behind the serving counter-which was always a difficult one for me. I could not see the items, and the staff would have most likely been too busy to help, resulting in an awkward moment. I ordered what turned out to be a delicious BLTA (a BLT with avocado). She helped me kindly, as if she knew I had vision problems, but we never discussed how she knew.

When connecting from Charlotte to Greensboro I was now on my own, as Cerise only flew as far as Charlotte. I moved up closer to the overhead departure screen than the crowd around me, as I usually did. I still could not see the concourse or gate number for Greensboro. I could make out the G's and could distinguish Green Bay from Greensboro as words, but I could not make out the concourse letter or gate number to the right of the destination names. I waited, hoping it would come into focus, but this time it did not. A young boy and his mother had also come up close to the screen to find their connection. Playfully I asked the young boy if he could spot the Greensboro information, as if it were a game. He did, and his mother confirmed the information for me. I was thankful. As they walked away she turned and took a good look at me to try to figure out why I asked them, and they were off, as was I. At Hema's prompting, I just needed to get more comfortable dealing with these issues and asking for help. I was trying.

At the conference the previous year, people at the Disability Issues Caucus business meeting were excited about the accessibility of the relatively new conference center at the Vegas Hotel. This was understandable given the complexity of the spaces at the Chicago Hilton—which had narrow cluttered corridors, and difficult twists and turns in parts of that conference space. Dodging people and the water dispensers placed in those narrow halls, was a challenge for some. I was curious how well things would be sign-posted and organized at the Vegas conference. It turned out to be a mixed experience. Although the main hallway to the conference area was flat and wide, a positive for the wheelchair bound, the conference facility was a struggle for me. The conference room signage was high overhead, and small, and therefore difficult to see. The conference presentation rooms themselves were dingy, making any paper notes I used a struggle to see.

After my paper presentation on blindness and teaching, in a Disability Issues Caucus panel, I chatted with the panel chair, Brian, a wheelchair bound colleague. We began by chatting about the panel. He was pleased at the "positive frame" of my paper, stating that it was good to hear a paper that portrayed the positive side of life of the disabled. I was pleased that the panel actually led to an interesting discussion of campus accessibility issues and challenges. We began by sharing perspectives on the conference hotel. I told him I was a "low vision" person, and that I found the lobby and conference rooms too dimly lit to be comfortable. He seemed to warm to me after I identified myself as a low vision person. He described how arduous of a journey it was from his room to the conference facility, and the carpet meant there was no momentum and he pushed all that way. I joked that it must be like moving through grass for him, and we shared a laugh as he agreed. He relayed an extraordinary story of another elderly wheelchair user who had actually taken a cab from the hotel lobby round the back of the hotel to the nearest conference area door. We both paused momentarily to ponder the scale of the place, and the bizarre and unfortunate image of the cab ride between two parts of the same hotel. The subtext of our conversation—we were people making the best of where we found ourselves, our struggles largely unnoticed by the crowds of conference participants who typically bustled quickly by with cell phones and Starbucks cups in hands.

Transitioning back to the campus issues in our conversation, while linking to "low vision" issues, he shared a story of a colleague who struggled every early morning with a security key pad which he had to use to gain access to his work area on campus. It reminded me momentarily of Hema's old apartment complex, and the difficulty I had punching the correct security code at night through my car window.

"If only they had a backlit key pad he would probably be ok"! I offered.

"Yes! That would really help" he responded. We saw important details that others do not notice.

I was curious about how Brian used classroom technology, so I asked him specifically about his experiences using media carts in classrooms. He smiled and said definitively, "They are completely inaccessible to me!"

He went on to explain by graphically acting how he would have to use his phone camera to relay down to himself what is up on the screen of the media cart computer. I paralleled his description by acting out how closely I would have to get to the glass case to see the computer screen inside when I used media carts—my face pressed up against the glass. We shared the joke again of a common struggle in a world that does not fully focus on accessibility for everyone. Classroom technology was a long way from being accessible for disabled and low vision instructors at many campuses. Rather, implicit in the design of classroom media, is an assumption that instructors stand at a particular height, and can see clearly down to the small computer screen in the cart. We moved to the corridor outside the room and chatted a while longer. Shortly after we said our farewells, I felt guilty that I did not offer to help him on the arduous journey back to the lobby. It felt awkward to offer help in that moment, as it was difficult to know how such an offer might be construed. Perhaps I was overthinking it. Perhaps I should have at least walked back with him if we were going the same way.

Shortly after I got back home from the conference, on November 17th I received an email from Dad saying that we should not expect our inheritance any time soon as his check up in relation to his bladder cancer treatment had come back "negative." The doctor told him to come back in one year. I know this was great for him to hear. He had become tired and annoyed at the constant follow up appointments, and the irritating waste of time spent waiting that came with them. I emailed right back to say congratulations, and that hearing the statement "come back in one year" was always good to hear. I understood. I had enjoyed a yearly check-up for my eyes for the last couple of years during a stable period, and it was good to see him put the disease and worry aside as much as possible. He was cycling out of a worry period, just as I was cycling back into one. My new appointment schedule was compressed to three months, as his expanded to a year.

Invitations to Share

In the middle of December, I got an email from Lea at LMRI, asking if I would answer some questions regarding my experience of living with MacTel. They were beginning an initiative to post "profiles" of patients on their web-site as an information resource for other patients. I was thrilled to be asked. She asked about doing an interview over the phone, which I said was ok, but that I would rather answer questions in written form so that I could think about them a bit. Within a day or two she emailed me some questions for me to respond to, and I began to think about what aspects of my experience might be of interest and use to other patients. It was an exciting opportunity to share my experiences, and I devoted substantial time to writing and editing my responses over the long winter break.

Later that month, the MacTel Facebook site posted a call for participants for the genetic study that I was part of. They wanted cousins who had MacTel, giving them enough genetic differences within close familial pairings to help isolate key genes. It affirmed Dr. John's explanation and, perhaps, helped clarify why David was not being sought after for his genes as much as we expected.

For New Year's we had developed a tradition of going to the beach. This time we went to North Myrtle beach as Hema wanted to try a condo resort complex her friend Mini recommended. She did all of the driving, insisting on it even though I offered to do some. She was tired and in pain from a stiff neck and back. On our way back we added an hour to the trip by driving over to see a retired colleague, Joyce, who was now living at Holden beach. She was a widow now and moved there for a change, and to be close to her son and two sisters. It was great to see her, but it added to Hema's driving, and it was a long day for her as she was still in some pain. The next morning she was up early and off back to work. When she got home that night we argued and irritated each other. Before falling asleep she cried and hugged me. She was just so tired she was overly emotional. I could have driven some of the way, but she insisted on doing it all for us.

After much re-reading and editing of my answers to the LMRI interview questions, on January 5th I emailed my responses to Leah. I tried to capture my story briefly, and outlined some concrete advice for fellow MacTel patients. This would go onto the LMRI website sometime soon. I hoped they liked the information, and I hoped that I had not written too much. She wrote back the next day to say that she thoroughly enjoyed reading the answers, and that she thought the information would be beneficial to other MacTel patients. I was very glad to hear it. A day or two later, once the permission form was signed and returned to them, the answers—capturing my experience of the first four and a half years in a few pages—now belonged to the LMRI. I was thrilled to provide this information, and hoped that good things would come from it. I gave them permission to use my full name, so that people would easily be able to contact me in response to my "profile" if they wanted to.

On January 10th David posted a picture of some geese in the dim light of an early winter morning in England, at his local pond. The caption with the picture read, "I'm liking my camera Christmas present … my local ducks looking a bit spooky." I resisted the urge to joke about how his ducks were actually geese. This would have been an exploitation of the moment, and he would have likely taken it the wrong way. Rather, I simply "liked" the posting and silently empathized with his love of the simple visuals of nature that surrounded him. He was enjoying what he *could* see in the same way that I did, as I also walked around the pond where I lived, several thousand miles away. Again, silently, I hoped that he would use the camera to revel in the beauty around him, shape, form, and color—to savor the simple visual moments of *life* just as I was.

Over a marvelous dinner of Ash and rice pilaf—Azerbaijani classics, at the Askerov's one cold night over MLK weekend Ali slipped into the conversation the question, "How well can you see?"

I wasn't sure how to respond as I was not sure in what context he meant it. Quickly he filled in with another question, "Can you see to the end of the kitchen?" He asked, searching for a point of reference ahead of me.

"Yes, yes!" Of course I could. It was only a few feet away.

"Well I have seen you a couple of times at the park and I recognized you from quite a distance, but I don't think you recognized me so quickly!"

"Yes! I remember recognizing you just as you were about to pass me." I replied.

I think he was trying to understand why I did not recognize him, and I was hoping he was not misunderstanding my limitations as a personal slight. It would have been easy for him to think I was only recognizing him after he spoke to me. I do not think he was thinking this but, to clarify, I offered: "The eye condition I have means that sometimes I can't recognize faces very well, even when people are close up."

"Ahh!" He replied and, I think to make me feel better, added that he thinks his vision is also declining.

"Anyway, at the park I am so focused on walking, I don't often really look at people, especially when it's cold." I acted out my walking style on a cold day, head down and arms swinging, making it reasonable to expect that I might not notice someone, even if I knew them.

"I am the same way," he added-affirming our similarity. Then the conversation moved on to other things that included our wives.

My car, being a 2000 model, was by now a solid 15–16 years old. It still looked good on the outside, but it was definitely showing wear and tear on the inside. Hema began to push me to think about buying a newer one. I did not want payments, and I only really drove a few miles a day—to the office and back. So I resisted. She was having one of her "intuitive feelings" that I was supposed to go with, this time that I would be in for some expensive repairs soon. She may well have been right, and I had not had any car expenses in a long time so perhaps I was due. But I still resisted. Again I thought to myself, I did not know how long I would be driving, and I did not want to jump into a loan at this point with so many other expensive projects around the house in motion. She pressed me into discussing what I would like to drive if I were to change cars. Perhaps a Mini Cooper, I offered. It would be good for the quick ten minutes to the office every day, and the hatch-back would give us some much needed variety from her similar four door saloon car. The hatch-back would enable us to pick up home décor items without asking friends with SUV's or trucks for help, as we had done recently with some new cabinets. Within minutes of the discussion, she had narrowed the search online to ones available in our area, and wanted to know which one I would like to test drive! Somehow I pushed the moment off against the many other things we were mired with at the moment, and things diffused away into other topics.

On January 22nd I got an email from the interim chair of Peace and Conflict Studies to tell me that our GA, Derrick, who had been helping me with all of the nit-picky, and for me sight intensive, detailed copyediting work for the two books, was being reassigned by her to help with her research while Tom was away on his Fulbright to Germany. It was a bad start to Friday. I was angry and a little afraid. He had helped me enormously to get the manuscripts to this point. Tom had done very little on either book, so I was now essentially alone in managing the details for both books, which were already behind schedule.

On that same day, I got a reminder from Wake Forest Baptist that my three month follow-up appointment was due the following Friday January 29th. It caught Hema by surprise, and she groaned, when I mentioned it the next day. She had missed several days of work with bronchitis last week, and also missed Friday due to winter storm Jonas, which left us snowbound in the house for the whole weekend. She was becoming acutely conscious of needing to get back in the flow of making deals at work. She was doing a search with the CEO, at his request, and the pressure to perform was on. To avoid a stressful moment, I suggested we ask our friend Deepak to drive me there. He had volunteered a while ago in the eventuality that I needed a ride and Hema could not get off work. He had flexible time, but still, this was a major favor. I was trepidant as Hema had always taken me to Wake, and it would be a whole morning just to take me for a check-up. But she made the call to Deepak, and the agreement to take me was set. I had to be at Janeway Tower by 8:30 am, and Deepak was not a morning person. I felt a little guilty, but tried not to feel like a "bother" as my mother would say. Hopefully, things were stable, and I would be back to six months or even a year. *Hopefully*.

The Three Month Follow-Up and Beyond

I jumped out of bed at six that morning as if I had an international flight to catch. "Let's get there and see what the deal is" I thought to myself, now a veteran of many such appointments. Hema dropped me off at Deepak and Asha's house who were there to greet us, offering us Chai, which we did not have time for. Hema had to rush to work for a company photograph at eight o'clock sharp, and she did not want to miss it. Asha had put together a snack bag of homemade banana nut break and bananas. One small bag each for both Deepak and myself, contained in a brown lunch bag which he carried to the car for us. It was so thoughtful and cute. Deepak made his usual morning power shake, which he would have in the waiting room while he made work related calls and waited for me. Thoughtfully, they had melded their familiar routines into and around the trip to Wake Forest. Deepak and I made it there on time and, as my number was called, I left him to his professional calls in a cozy corner of the spacious and bright waiting room.

At area D, I was ushered into an examining room and given the familiar, and dreaded, letter test. I think I came out ok. I answered the usual questions: Had I travelled out of the country recently? Had I noticed any changes? The stinging dilation drops were dropped into my eyes, and I was left to wait. Then the technician told me, just before she left, that I would first meet one of their fellows. I asked what a fellow was, for clarity. Then I would meet with Dr. John and a student. He was introducing them to their first look at eyes impacted by MacTel. Mine! After what seemed like a long wait, the fellow entered. He asked me a couple of standard questions and noted, out loud, that it had been three months since the last examination. He proceeded to look into my eyes at close range with a lighted device. After a few moments he announced assuredly, "The bleeding you had last time is all gone. No sign of it!"

I was thrilled.

"That is a *very* good sentence to hear!" I replied, as he pulled away to write some notes on the computer. He told me that six months until the next appointment would be fine, unless I noticed any changes. I was so relieved. When he left, I texted Hema that all was well, and waited for Dr. John and his student to come. Then I sat back in the chair and just closed my eyes for a moment and relaxed in gratitude. The news could have been very different. Those dreaded dots could have been there, they could have gotten worse, they could have caused swelling that would have necessitated an injection, and a follow up in just a month. But this was the best news possible, and I savored its meaning for me as I sat alone in the big examining chair. Six months would be all the way until sometime in July I calculated, which seemed like such a long way off on a frosty morning at the end of January. Although I do not think he minded, I would not need to inconvenience Deepak again for a whole morning spent taking me to my appointment. Surely by July Hema would be able to take me again. Perhaps moving forward I would rotate through various people, in order to spread out the burden of driving me there.

Dr. John entered and introduced a young man to me as a fourth year medical student, and introduced me to him as Dr. Kellett! He wanted the young medical student to take a close look at my optic nerves, and left while he set up to do this. The aspiring Doctor fiddled a little uncomfortably with the apparatus that was in front of my face. I even tried to help him adjust it, but he got the hang of it and managed to take a good look into my eyes. Participating in the teachable moment, I asked him: "So tell me, what can you see?"

"The optic nerve looks fine, but I can see the damaged areas around the fovea—the center of vision" he said.

"More on the right eye right?" I asked, encouraging him to expand on his observation.

"Yes a little more on the right eye." He responded.

"Is this the first time you have seen eyes with MacTel?" I inquired.

"Yes it is … first time."

Dr. John entered and we caught up quickly. He restated the good news that everything looked stable, and the need to come back in six months. We chatted about my profile being used by the LMRI, and he was pleased. He shared that he was starting a collaborative research project with an economist on the impact of socio-economic status on diabetes related eye problems, and I encouraged him with the project. We wrapped up and firmed up my interest in coming to speak to his students this summer. As we left the examination room I joked,

> "You will have your grant and now you just need your new building!" referencing back to a conversation last time about his dream of a new eye-center at Wake Forest. "Yes, you're going to help me with that right?" he replied, as we shook hands to say a final farewell. Momentarily I was puzzled. Was he expecting a donation from me? Would $50 make a difference I thought to myself ironically? Then, as I walked away in the direction of the place to make my next appointment, I remembered our conversation on the last visit where he said he would want input on the design from actual eye patients. He was firming up his invitation, and I appreciated it, albeit silently.

Deepak was surprised to see me so soon. I had some of Asha's banana nut bread, as he finished his breakfast shake. We headed back to the car and, as we pulled up to the pay booth, he refused to let me pay for the parking. There was no need for him to cover parking costs as well, but he insisted. We were back to Greensboro in good time and, as he dropped me off, I told him that Hema and I wanted to take him and Asha out for dinner as a thank you. His parting words as I got out of his car at our house were,

> "That's not necessary. Our friendship goes way beyond that. But, we will get together when you are both feeling better."
> "Thank you!" I replied, simply, touched by the warm generosity and kindness of his friendship. Then, as I closed the car door, I quickly headed up the driveway for the dim light of the inside of the house. It was a bright sunny day, and I was still widely dilated.

Hema returned home later that evening, and presented me with her detailed performance evaluation. She had received a very good review and left it on the coffee table for me to read. It was too dark in the room for me to read, so I took it to my desk and sat down with it. She had established herself well and everyone who was part of the review said how well she had started at CAI, and how promising her future looked with the company. It was a moment of symmetry in our good news that was a long time coming, and all the more worth savoring. My eyes appeared stable, and her career was taking off. On top of this, after what had been a long drawn out process, we also now had our new beautiful countertops installed. We could begin reorganizing from chaos closer to order in our small home. We also had both just about gotten over illnesses that had made the last week or so a misery—pneumonia for me, and bronchitis for Hema. So, things had come together in a good moment here on Friday evening. We celebrated with a drive out to Taaza restaurant in Burlington where we had had our wedding reception two and a half years ago. It was always good to go there and reconnect a little with that history, and with each other, after a busy week.

During spring break, which was the second week of March for me, I heard from my old friend Joe. I had not heard from him in a while. We had recently reconnected and restarted our friendship after a few years of him disappearing upon retirement to Flagstaff Arizona. It was unusual for him to initiate an email sequence. Usually I had to make contact first, which often became annoying. On March 9th he sent me an email entitled, "How are you, Pete?" In the email he passed on a reference to a BBC online news item on stem cell applications to eye conditions. He closed with, "I remember you had mentioned that stem cell surgery might be in your future. Any news?" I was glad to hear from him, and recognized that he had thought about me when the story popped up on the BBC website, and he remembered my eye condition. His inquiry about my news was a first in several years. He was using the story as a way in to firm up renewed contact, and to show that he cared enough to connect, remember, and inquire.

I wrote back with a thanks and clarified that I kept up with the research, and that I had registered with the MacTel project which might help me down the line. I wished him an early happy birthday, which was four days away. He wrote back to say that his wife was visiting a friend who had recently suffered a major stroke and who was partially paralyzed as a result. He was not expecting a big day of celebrations for his birthday was the subtext. The other subtext was that we were entering a period of life where anything could happen.

"Yep, we're in that cohort where shit like this happens. Where did all that time go, man.?" He wrote. We had been friends for thirty-five years and, although it may have seemed that we had not changed that much, we had, and life had. We were both now solidly in our 50s. A lot of time had slipped away.

I wrote right back to say how awful that was and that, "Yep, you never know" I went on to explain that our worry here is that neither Hema nor myself have any family here to rely on down the road, but that we did not want to live in England or India. He wrote right back, "Same thing here, Pete. Wouldn't want to live in Italy or England."

We were creating an important point of parallel experience—a comparison of our similar life stages through our health talk, and related worries. We were affirming something in common, something on which to base our renewing friendship as we edged well into middle-age and beyond.

· 20 ·

SOCIAL MEDIA, CONNECTEDNESS, STRUGGLE AND HOPE

Around the beginning of February, I wanted to return to the online world of information and connection that The LMRI was actively creating through its regular social media postings and invitations. I realized I had not made time to participate, even though I thought their social media based information was an important innovation, with patient's needs centrally in mind. I just had not made the effort to make the time. So, I looked back over their Facebook postings for ways that I might begin to participate more actively, and maybe even get to know some fellow patients around the world. There were many postings that related to medical breakthroughs, and I noticed there was a very active construction of hope. Innovations and breakthroughs in medical research into medications and genetic techniques were a consistent theme for postings. Collectively the posts constructed the hope that a cure was on its way for many eye diseases. As I looked through them all for the last few months I could feel the hope, but also I wondered about hope gaps and hope fatigue. Were all of these inspiring research leads adding up to much of anything for ordinary people with MacTel? Over time I noticed that I skipped over many of the postings that had this theme of being "on the verge of a major breakthrough" especially when the posts did not relate directly to MacTel. Other types of postings, more realistic or experiential ones, were harder to find, and got less attention. For example, I noticed one posting tucked away somewhere in winter from a woman who was sharing that her condition had accelerated over the course of only one year, leaving her disabled. There were very few replies or likes on her posting. I felt sad for her. Perhaps people just did not know what to say. Other postings encouraged connecting with fellow patients, but I had missed these by several months and it felt awkward to suddenly pop up announcing myself. So I did not initiate anything, or respond to any of the postings, except to like a few of them that were particularly relevant to MacTel related research or experience.

One evening in my graduate class called Positive Communication Research we were talking about communication at the end of life as the topic for the evening. I had several online sites that I wanted to show them, including Artful Ashes, where people had the ashes of loved ones integrated into art glass objects that spoke to our discussion of aesthetics and positive post-end of life communication. I decided that tonight was the night I would use the media cart in the room, and run through a few sites for them. This was something I had avoided for several years since my eye problems began, as the media carts were a challenge. The laptop inside the case was small and difficult to see, but I was determined to use presentational technology this semester. I practiced on the machine during the afternoon when the classroom was empty. It was easy to use, and I felt confident that all would go well. As the pair of graduate students introducing the topic finished, I jumped up and announced that I would show them some online information. I began well, showing them a book series by Peter Lang that provided some background to the Life-span approach of the topic. I told them there was a surprise and, as I scrolled down, they spotted the information on a book by their graduate director, Loreen Olson. A collective cheer went up for Loreen. All was going well, until I tried to locate the Artful Ashes page. Somehow I clicked on the wrong thing and ended up looking at Gmail login instead of Google. They began coaching me as I could not tell the difference. The login logo for both Gmail and Google looked too similar to me at the size they were on the screen. Instead of closing the correct page, somehow I had gone in the wrong direction and they could see up on the screen that I was not doing well. I tried to stay calm and just told them, "Sorry, I can't see the screen …"

They were kind enough to supportively coach me back to where I needed to re-login, as embarrassing as it was for me. I found the Artful Ashes page and showed them a You Tube video about how the art glass with ashes inside are made. As I was embarrassed because of my struggles, I did not look at them while I was searching around, but I stuck with it and did not give up. For that I was proud of myself, but it was embarrassing to struggle in front of an audience. I think it helped that I had been open with them during the semester about my condition, and in sharing my article about end of life conversations with pal Bud Goodall (Kellett, 2013). They knew I was not incompetent, but rather that the inaccessible technology was the issue. At the break I talked to Maria, my deaf interpreter student, and we talked about how classroom technology here, and other things at UNCG, are not accessible for disabled people. I had given it a try, with mixed success, but I did try, and at least we saw the sites I had wanted to show them.

Online Encouragement, Connection, and Hope

The skies were brightening, the days were getting longer, and I could feel spring rising around me and through me. As I left my evening class that Wednesday night after my technology issues, it was warm and still a slight hint of daylight lit the high spring sky. It was such a relief to have light to drive home by and not just the scant street lights. I had made it through the dark part of the year without incident and with reasonable confidence that I could drive safely, within reason, until May and the end of the academic year—a minor milestone for me.

Things around the yard began to bloom again. The fruit trees looked vigorous and healthy after a fairly mild winter. This year it looked like we would get lots of figs, Hema and I assured one Saturday as we looked around at things. There were tiny figs starting to appear on the long, elegant, flexible branches. There were the small buds of densely folded up leaves appearing at the end of each branch. I could see them all—budding figs, budding leaves—budding and blooming was everywhere, and I loved it. I was thankful and I was happy to be here in this life that had been so good to me. I knew the onslaught of eye fatigue was about to become difficult, as grading started to mount up for several hours each day, but the end of the academic year was starting to also bud into view with its sweet scent of freedom blooming and wafting in the distance, just over the hill and round the bend.

In March, I was coming up on the due date for my five year performance review and, as I began to pull my materials together, I was confident that I would have a good rating. Just as importantly, for me, I had begun talks around campus about creating a disability studies program, and several people were interested in collaborating. Celia Hooper the Dean of Health and Human

Sciences was particularly interested, noting that many of the programs in her unit would be interested in this idea. The provost was supportive, writing right back after I contacted her with the ideas to offer support. She even requested that I keep her posted on developments, which I did. Perhaps this would breathe new life into my time at UNCG which had grown somewhat stale and mechanical—especially in my home department of Communication Studies. Perhaps it would be a valuable addition to campus as much as it might be for me personally and professionally—focusing people that I, as yet, did not know very well, on teaching and learning about disability as a common interest.

Hema frequently assured me that she would be happy to leave Greensboro if a good job came up somewhere else for me. However, I feared my ability to get to know another city in terms of getting around and driving safely and confidently in an unfamiliar place. In Greensboro, I knew most of the streets as second nature. I did not voice this to her because I did not know how she would react. She did not like fearful reactions to life decisions. I think this was primarily because she perceived her father to have been dominated too much by fear in his decision making, and she did not want to see the same thing in me. She also did not like me clinging to familiar patterns as if stuck in a comfort zone. This was boring to her. But it nagged at me as a reason to stay here in Greensboro. This place was in many ways a comfort zone, our adopted home town, but it worked well for me as such. I knew how to get around and do the basics here, and I knew enough people who could help me with the rest if I needed help. It was a familiar place which did not produce many significant challenges in living here. Yet those new challenges, and the opportunities that came with a change of location, were what Hema craved in our life. She wanted to be out of this comfort zone, as she did almost any comfort zone, while I relied on it for peace of mind. My thinking was that living in this comfortable place meant I could focus more on my writing and less on dealing with the additional challenges of a new location. Her thinking, I believe, was that a new place would bring new life to work and the rest of our life together.

April 1st was a big day for me. In the morning I was meeting with the Disability Studies Committee. We had more people joining the group and bringing many years of experience working in the world of disabilities or, as Phelps from Peacehaven Farm cleverly suggested, "diffabilities." It was a good humored and productive meeting, but I also felt a little out of my area of expertise. I was surrounded by professionals and academics who were vastly more knowledgeable than me on the topic. I said as much as we went around the room with brief introductions. About half way through the meeting I also felt another group member trying to nudge for control of the meeting. I saw the usual tactics: suggesting things to discuss that were already on the agenda I had emailed around. Acting like things were not moving as well as they would if they were in charge, and that things were their idea when they were not. Usual academic meeting dynamics, and not a big deal, but I really did not enjoy it. I had not been in charge of anything for several years since stepping off as Head of my department, and the familiar feeling of trying to run a meeting with someone else jockeying to be in control, gave me a feeling that I did not miss at all. After the meeting, I thought about suggesting that someone else leads the process. After all, the minor in Disability Studies would be housed in a different department, in a different academic unit and, as long as the program was created, I did not need to be in charge of it.

That afternoon, I emailed my graduate student, Maria, to thank her for coming to the meeting. She wrote a lovely message back encouraging me, and reframing my newness to the field of Disability Studies as an asset.

My Online Interview Narrative

That night was the first "First Friday" of the season in downtown Greensboro. Hema and I and Deepak went downtown and walked around in the blustery but warm spring evening. There was music and good spirits in the air. Shops and coffee bars were open late and we all enjoyed the evening out. Later that night, as I lay in bed and checked email and Facebook before going to sleep, I saw a posting from the MacTel group. Someone called Marge was inviting us to check out the new information on the LMRI website: "Hi Folks-this is Marge again. I had a nice surprise tonight as I decided the check out the Lowy Medical Research Institute's website since I hadn't been on it for a week or two. Much to my surprise they had updated the website and there is some new information. They have even included the option where you can increase/decrease the size of the text! Please be sure to check out all of the sections, especially the 'Diagnosing MacTel' and the link below 'Patient Perspectives.'"

Could this be the part of the website that would feature my interview, I wondered to myself? As I lay there, I decided I did not want to click on it in case it was a disappointment, being about something else. The meeting today had disappointed me enough, and I was too tired to follow the link. So I left the page unopened but on my IPad for me to look at in the morning.

The next morning I opened up the page and clicked on it. It opened directly to my interview questions and answers (http://www.lmri.net/pete-kellett/). I was thrilled to see it finally posted to the website. As I showed Hema, she was curious to know if mine was the only one posted. It seemed that mine was the first to be posted, but I assumed—and hoped—there would be many more to come. This lifted my day from the very beginning, and put me in a wonderful Saturday morning mood. LMRI was really trying to be a resource, and I was glad to be part of it.

As I scrolled down the post I saw that several people had liked the posting and link by Marge. I was particularly heartened to read that several people found the new information, of which my story was a small but meaningful part, useful. Beth posted: "I have just more about MacTel 2 reading the updates web site (sic) than I have in the 4½ years since diagnosis. I have been going to one of the 'premier' eye centers in the world and haven't gleaned as much knowledge as I just did in the last 20 minutes. Thank you for posting."

Similarly, Michelle posted: "Newly diagnosed at 39 yrs. Learned so much when I read this. And in South Africa it is even more unknown disease. Thank you."

I was filled with encouragement that perhaps my story had helped. Of course, I did not know exactly what part of the information she found useful. It could have been the information they had posted about diagnosis and symptoms. But whatever it was, this was a very positive moment. The information was being read and valued because it was designed to be helpful, and people were finding it so.

I commented on Marge's post: "Very glad to have some of my experiences posted to the site! Please add more everyone." I encouraged.

Someone from the LMRI liked my post later that day, as they did all of the posts by people responding to the website information. They were glad to see the enthusiastic, if small, response. There were a few comments and, at that time, 16 likes. A couple of days later I got a notification that two people liked my comment, which meant a lot to me.

Marge herself completed the short list of comments under her post with a thank you to the Lowy family, who were integral to the existence of the LMRI, and to everyone involved. This was a nice touch that acknowledged, in part, that they were going out of their way to be an information resource, a source of connections between patients and, importantly, a source of hope for a cure: "I would just like to add and I've said it many times before-a BIG thank you to the Lowy Family and all of the researchers and folks working to find a cure for us!! We finally have hope and for that we are grateful to all of you!!"

Later that day I looked through the new information on diagnosis and also found it useful as a central resource on symptoms and diagnostics. The "Patient Perspectives" section did have a text magnifier which some on Facebook had referred to with gratitude. The introduction read as follows:

> "MacTel is a relatively rare disease. As such, there is limited information available to patients who have been recently diagnosed and are looking to learn about MacTel. The patient perspectives featured here are an opportunity for people with Mactel to share their stories of living with the disease, and how they have adapted to deal with changes to their vision."

There was a link alongside an invitation, "If you would like to share your MacTel story, please contact us." I was warmly heartened to see that the LMRI were approaching this as a narrative sharing opportunity. There was now, in their wording, such a thing as a "MacTel story" and the Institute was interested in soliciting and sharing them with anyone visiting the LMRI website. The fact that mine was the first to be featured, was an added thrill for me. I had asked them to include my name with the interview, which they did, and I hoped that I might hear from people who read my interview, and wanted to share experiences. I did not hear from anyone directly, but that was fine. The information was useful, and this was just the beginning.

I sent a message to Alie, my former graduate student and co-author of a recent book chapter, to ask if she had sent anything to NCA for next year, and to ask how she was doing. She wrote back with a long message about her post-partum issues and that she was going to group therapy several times a week. She affirmed that it has strengthened her interest in researching support related to health, which I was glad that she would be pursuing in her Ph.D. program. I responded that sometimes our research topics choose us, and to hang in there. I relayed to her that the LMRI has featured some of my story and that hopefully both of our stories would have an impact on people in their own ways. I was encouraging her that our parallel but different health issues might have positive value to others. I hoped she would continue journaling her experience, and that she would recover soon. She wrote back asking for a link to the interview. She asked to keep in touch and that she enjoyed hearing from me. It was a delight to me to keep in touch with students like Alie in this way, and to continue to have a positive relationship long after class is over.

She wrote back a day or so later to ask if I would help her if, at some point in the future, she turns her journaling of her post-partum experience into a book. At the end of her email she added that she had read my interview and that it was "Nice!" I was grateful for the encouraging feedback. In response, I encouraged her to work on a couple of publications based on her experiences in order to establish her voice on the topic. I believed that, down the road, she would turn this into something very valuable for other women with the same difficult experience.

I received an email from Lea at LMRI to tell me that my interview was now on their website. I already knew, but I was pleased to hear from her. She also indicated that they would add another interview in a few weeks, which was great. Even more significant, they would add a "Clinicians Perspective" soon. Perhaps this would lead to some positive developments in mutual understanding between health care providers, patients, and researchers. The information and communication sharing across all of us would be exciting to see emerge on their website, and I wondered if more face to face discussions and collaborations might be nurtured in the near future. I was thrilled to be part of this even in a very small way.

One evening I logged into my Wake Forest portal and left a message for Dr. John that my interview was featured on the new "Patient Perspectives" page on the LMRI web site. The next day (4/5/2016) he wrote back:

> "Hi Pete,
> Thank you so much for sharing. I have a deeper appreciation for your experience after reading your interview. On another note, do you work for the local NPR station? I swear I hear your voice some mornings on the radio.
> Vishak"

I wrote a quick note back to let him know that they would be adding a "Clinicians Perspectives" page soon, and that it might be a useful resource for his students given that the LMRI would be representing both sides of the health care process and experience. I also clarified that I did not work for the radio station, but that I hoped whomever it was sounded more intelligent than I would on the radio!

I sent the link to my interview to Dr. Rosenfeld and Cristy Lage-Rodriguez at Bascom Palmer at Miami University to let them know part of my story was now featured. I wanted to thank them for being part of my story, which they had been for my official diagnosis and donation of genetic sample for the clinical study that my genes were now part of. Cristy responded within an hour and wrote, "Thank you for being part of this global effort!"

I was pleased and proud to have part of my story featured, and I wanted people to read it. I sent the link to my blind former student and friend Kolby, who wrote right back to say thanks for sending her the link. She was busy as a court reporter but said she would love to catch up soon and introduce me to her new assistance dog. She asked me if I were still teaching at UNCG, which surprised me but I realized we had not met in a year or so. Perhaps we could meet on campus again soon, and have a walk round with her new dog.

On April 11th I got an email from Alie to say that today was her last day of group therapy for her post-partum support and recovery process. She described the day as "bittersweet." It occurred to me that so much of all of our health related experiences are bittersweet. The joy of a new child, and the choking fog of post-partum depression. Support that warms us, holds us close, and lifts us, only for us to be weaned off it so soon. A day or so later, she affirmed her newfound commitment to channeling her experiences into writing. She was making plans to meet with a faculty member next week who might be a good fit for her as an advisor. I looked her up on the website and was very impressed by her blossoming early career. She looked like a rising star, and I was glad that Alie had found someone. I knew they would be a good fit.

A day later she would appear to bounce back from the bittersweet feelings, and begin the act of love that I too had been engaging in, that is writing it all down for herself and, perhaps, for others. She messaged: "My goal today is to write out all of my feelings and experiences from the past few months … sort of a 'brain dump' so I don't forget or lose details as I continue to recover and the experience becomes more distant."

I knew just where she was. But I also knew that this would be something that would engage her for much more than a day as a "brain dump." If her experience paralleled mine, it would engage her most days that the experience was real and present to her. I hoped that the journaling would help her each day, and build into a fascinating story from the entries of each day as they connected together into a fuller story of recovery.

She affirmed: "My plan is to study social support and its connection to health—individual and relational. This experience has me wanting also to look at social support and mental health specifically because I think it is an area that is often overlooked when 'health' is mentioned, but is extremely important."

She went on to thank me for my continued support.

Through her emails over these few days, it seemed that she was recovering before my eyes. One day she was letting go of group therapy. The next she was beginning to write the experience, and make plans to meet with someone who might supervise a research agenda with her on this and related topics. I was thrilled to see this taking shape over a few emails, and I planned to continue to encourage her in this direction, however I could. This was a year full of encouragement and, happily, I was part of it in various ways.

· 21 ·

TOWARDS THE END OF YEAR FIVE

The Impact of Fatigue

The end of April and beginning of May brought crippling eye fatigue for me from reading and grading papers and exams. My eyes were so tired by the end of those long days of grading that I felt like keeping them closed in the evenings, even as we watched television. Eye fatigue made my brain tired, and it seemed to creep outwards from my eyes to the rest of my body, dragging everything downward and inward until grading was over. I was supposed to review papers for the Bud Goodall & Nic Trujillo award set up in their honor, but I opened the list and stopped in my tracks. I just could not read any more pages of print. I had to tell the chair of the committee to go with the other judges' rankings as I just could not do it. Bud had supported me so much as he was dying a few years ago but, with regrets, I could not repay the favor this time. I also had to put off reviewing papers for the Conflict and Peace Division for NCA for the same reason, but resolved to do them before the 11th as I had been granted an extension by the division chair. Finally, I finished grading and I sat through our department graduation knowing that it was all over again until next academic year. Freedom, relief, rest, and other positives swirled around in my mind, and I savored them. Yet I had set an intense writing program for the summer and only really took a weekend off before getting back to business.

On that weekend, in early May. The day of the Kentucky Derby, we went with Agnes and Bill to a baseball game in downtown Greensboro—the Grasshoppers versus a team from nearby Lexington. Although we sat very close up, on the third row behind home plate, I had a hard time seeing the ball, and an even harder time seeing the scoreboard. I figured out whether someone had been caught on the boundary or not by what they did next, and the sounds from the crowd, not by seeing the catches made or missed. I could not see the ball well at all. Watching the game through the safety netting did not help either. I found myself bored and increasingly weary, as the fatigue still lingering from grading week radiated from my eyes outwards to the rest of me. It was a lovely evening, and so good to see the young love of Agnes and Bill blossoming as they watched the game playfully. He explaining the game carefully to her, and she giggling as if she still did not really follow it. Hema did not know much about the game either, and struggled to figure out the scoreboard in order to explain to me where they were in terms of scores and innings. At one point Bill, perhaps sensing that we were bored, explained to us that they only played seven innings at this level. Only a short while later he had to correct himself and clarify that they played nine innings. I almost groaned in pain as he said this, as I knew we would be there for another half hour. Eventually we returned to our house as we had all driven in one car to the game.

To my surprise, and horror, as I was completely drained by this point, at 10:45 pm Hema insisted that they both come in for tea. After a little hesitation because of the lateness, they both agreed. I knew she was simply trying to hold onto Saturday—her favorite day, as Sunday meant starting to think about work again. The last few weeks had been stressful and difficult for her as she was working with a senior person who was negative, critical, and unfair, all things that made her freeze up and stress out. But how could she extend the evening further, knowing I was ready just to take my eyes to bed for the night? I was quietly furious, and went into the bathroom—tensing up my body into a silent scream of frustration before coming out into the kitchen, composed again, to help with the tea making. Soon she was coming back to life after the boring baseball game, and was in full conversational flow about her family and other favorite topics. I sat quietly drinking tea and trying not to appear rude to our guests, but I could not help thinking how selfish this was. When they finally left, I avoided lashing out, which was good for everyone, and I simply went off to bed, falling asleep as my head touched the pillow. She explained the next day that she just wanted to hold onto Saturday, as I had suspected, as it was her day away from anything work related. I understood enough not to make an issue of it, but it was an effort not to do so.

The Impact of Sharing Stories

In mid-May, I went to the LMRI website to forward the link to my interview to a couple of friends, Steve and Art, both of whom had followed this journey closely with me for almost five years now. I was pleased to see another interview loaded to the Patients Perspectives page. The interviewee had very similar experiences to mine, although she was never misdiagnosed as I had been. I was struck by her description of grieving when she was diagnosed. I too had gone through something like that, although I could not quite identify with the typical stages of anger and denial, and so on. Mine had been more like confusion and disappointment, followed by a resolve to adapt, with anger popping up throughout. But I could empathize as she described her children's inability to relate to her crying and grieving that followed her diagnosis. I too had been very afraid and sad, and found very little helpful information out there online during those early stages. I was heartened, also, by her insistence on making the positive turn towards adapting and making the most of life. Her adaptations and related frustrations were almost identical to mine, and I chuckled when she described how she had complained at her local Starbucks because they only had an overhead menu on the wall behind the counter—making it difficult to see. I had lived much the same story as she did. I knew that as this online information evolved to include more posted stories, it would be a very valuable resource, particularly for new patients. I wish there would have been a way to contact her, or at least "like" her narrative, or make a comment on it, but I noticed that she only had her first name listed, so it was unlikely that she wanted to be contacted.

Steve wrote a nice note back to me about my interview, saying how he forwarded it to Susan, his wife. As a therapist, there might be something she could learn from it. He was also kind enough to say that, although my sight was impaired, that I often "saw" more than most people. Perhaps this was a reference to the songs I had written for us to play together over the years. I was not sure, but it was a kind and generous word whatever it meant.

I read through my interview carefully to recall what I had shared. Finally, after it had been posted for a month or so, on May 16th, I messaged my brother, David, to suggest he read the interviews. I also encouraged him to share his own story so far with them. I do not really know why I held off from telling him sooner but, for some reason, as soon as there was another interview posted, I shared the site with him. Sending a link to a site featuring just my interview would somehow have been awkward. To my surprise, as I sat at my desk writing, my I-pad pinged with a message. It was David saying "Ok I will check it out." I was surprised that he responded so quickly, and hoped he would find the two interviews useful to read.

David wrote back again within an hour to say simply, "Good site" and to catch me up on the fact that they did finally take a genetic sample of his, so they had both of us now. He half joked that perhaps my contacts could help stimulate them to look into the genetics, as he did not have a lot of confidence in how organized the people were at his hospital. I understood his frustration given how long it took for them to take his sample, but the good news was that we were both finally in the genetic study sample. He did not say anything directly about my interview, which was odd, but not altogether surprising. I wrote back to clarify that I think they are looking for cousins, and other close but not identical relatives, for this stage of the genetic study. I ended by asking him how his vision was. He wrote back to say that his scans suggested that things were stable, and added that some days were better than others. He also said that it was a process of adapting, as mirrored in the two interviews posted so far on the Patients Perspectives page. I wrote back completing the brief interaction and to affirm his sentiment by saying simply: "Stability is good. Yes it seems to be tougher some times more than others."

For me, however, it was not so much days that were different, or better than other days, although the brightness of one day was much more difficult to navigate than the cooler gloom of another. For me, visual acuity varied by moments and this, I believed, was related to momentary changes in blood pressure—but I had no real substantiation for this idea. I did notice that if I suddenly got up from my desk at the office to walk to the restroom or to a meeting, this was when faces passing me in the corridor were difficult for me to recognize. Similarly, I also noticed that when I sat undisturbed at the computer screen for a while, I could focus well and things would be fine. But, if I got up and moved around, thus increasing blood pressure by activity, then my eyes were blurry and had to readjust back down to a stable state. I was not sure that this is what he meant, but this is what seemed to create variations for me. In fact, by way of an experimental illustration, half way through writing this paragraph, I got up to remove a peppermint tea bag from my cup so that my tea would not get bitter. As I returned from the kitchen and sat down to write again, the middle of my field of vision was gray and feint. Also, some of the letters on the screen page were distorted with some appearing much larger than others. So, to adjust, I found myself writing this moment while just looking down at the keys until my eyes settled back down. It took slightly less than a minute for my eyes to come back into balance.

I had all but given up on lapidary arts as a hobby, although I still clung to the equipment. I made plans to have a jeweler friend make a necklace for Hema consisting of some of the favorite stones I had cut over the years. It was ready just as our anniversary arrived on memorial-day weekend. It would be a poignant way for me to mark the end of something I had loved by having something made for Hema, which hopefully she would love.

A Weekend Away

In early June, we were invited to join Art and Jennifer in Wilmington for a weekend. They had rented a house for her 60th birthday getaway and her parents could not make the trip, so we joined them. Our weekend at the coast started badly. Hema drove, as usual. We were fine until close to Wilmington. Suddenly a missed exit, and an episode where our GPS would not cooperate, and we were adding an hour and a half onto an already long and dull drive. Tempers flared as frustrations boiled over. I wanted to get there. She wanted to get there. But we just could not seem to make the final turn to downtown. We kept ending up taking huge detours around the town. Several times we were close to downtown only to find ourselves being directed back out to I-40. Once we even started to head back towards Greensboro, courtesy of the GPS. At one point we pulled off into a scrappy neighborhood, lost. Hema turned to me as I complained and asked, "Well why don't you help?"

"Because I can't fucking see!" I replied, coming right back at her with explosive frustration. It was true, I could not help with road signs or street names in the dark, and I could not help much with the GPS on her small phone. I felt helpless and angry. But she was the one doing all of the work, and this, after a long and demanding week at work. She was exhausted and close to giving up. I told her that if we passed a hotel, we would stop and check in for the night. Somehow we got back on track after the outburst cleared the air a little, and we realized we just needed to keep getting closer to the lights of downtown. Either Jennifer or Art had given us bad directions—take the left fork, when it was actually the right. Once we tracked back and did this correctly, we were on Front Street, and almost there. Hema was very tired, but insisted on staying up to keep Jennifer company long into the night, and long after Art and I had both loped off to our beds.

The next morning I got up early and left Hema in peace to sleep in for some much needed rest. Jennifer is a late to bed, late to rise person, and we rarely saw her before 11 am. It was an enjoyable time together, but it was awkward accommodating and adjusting to everyone's sleep patterns. Art and I would rise early and meet on the front porch to talk and have breakfast. Hema would get up next. Then we would all wait for Jennifer to start the process of her getting up. It was a blazing hot and bright weekend, and I would have much preferred us getting up early and all going out for the morning to do things and explore. We could have walked around for a few hours, had a nice lunch somewhere, and then come back to rest inside when it was blazing hot and bright in the afternoon. As it turned out, we would hang around all morning, leave in time for a late lunch, and then start looking around town, right when I was dying to escape the blazing light. I wore a visor as well as clip-ons, but it did not help much. It was still the wrong place for me. As we wandered around shops, and between the vintage cars that were on show downtown, it was painful for me. I was used to morning activity and afternoon rest and retreat. On top of this Jennifer walked very slowly. It was frustrating, but here we were and we tried to have a good time. Late in our stay there was a nice conversational moment in the living room where Jennifer asked me about my eyes, and I explained the issues I had with bright light, and so on, but it did not change anything. During the summer, I had grown accustomed to controlling when I was outside, and when I was inside, but here I could not do that. I came home from the weekend wearier than when we left, and I know Hema did too. Monday morning, after driving back Sunday, was not a happy time. I was able to rest that day, but Hema was right back into the corporate rat race.

Learning From Others Stories

A third "Patient's Perspective" interview narrative appeared on the LMRI website in June, as did the first two "Clinician's Perspectives." The clinicians brought a fascinating "other side" to the information, with their own stories of how they came to work on this disease, and how their work is designed to impact understanding and treatment of MacTel. They affirmed, for me, the importance of the various forms of research. They also clarified what stage the main research projects were currently at, including the one in which David and I were subjects, and what had been discovered so far through the research. The interviews were fascinating as well as encouraging, and even comforting. One even spoke about the crucial patient practice of donating eyes—something I had committed to in Miami last year. I made a note to self to send Leah at LMRI a note to say how interesting I found the clinicians' interviews.

June, the third patient featured, shared many interesting experiences, particularly as someone with more advanced vision loss than I had. I could relate well to some of her struggles with reading, driving, and other everyday activities. I also caught a glimpse of life for someone with more advanced vision loss, and found her everyday practical adaptations fascinating. She had discovered, for example, that distinguishing shampoo from conditioner, and other similar containers, could be done by placing a rubber band on one of the containers—giving her a tactile clue to distinguish objects. I had noticed that shampoo and conditioners were often very similar, and the wording often small, so this made sense. She shared many other insights that showed her sense of humor, as well as her will to adapt, and stay independent as much as possible. She noted that she worried that she was becoming more dependent on her husband. Again, I could relate. I relied on Hema for so many things these days. The thing from her interview that really touched me, and that I found particularly fascinating, was her description of her being in "My Picasso stage." Faces were distorted—appearing to have one eyebrow, eyes out of normal alignment where one appears to be pulled into the other one, and a misshapen nose, as if she were looking at a Picasso painting. I could instantly relate to the period early on when my retinas were swelling, and bringing about gruesome facial distortion as I looked at people. To me, it felt more like a horror movie than a famous painting style. She may have had more time to adapt to the condition, and therefore find a more positive and playful image than the shock and horror I felt when I first saw distorted faces. It seemed from her narrative that this stage would return later due to more permanent blind spots and changes to the retina. She had found an elegant and evocative way to capture what it was like to see faces through her eyes. I admired her for this, as well as for the pluck with which she had adapted and moved on with her life as best she could.

Relationships, Meaning, and Life Together

After several months of success and relative happiness at work, Hema was assigned to a notoriously difficult project leader for two searches. It did not take long for him to be blitzing her with negative feedback and strangling her with micro-managing directives and critique. She never thrived in such difficult environments and, quickly, her enthusiasm for making deals was replaced by struggle, doubt, and stress. This brought on new self-doubts and much talk about what she wanted to do professionally. She began to distance her sense of self from what was expected at the search firm. She was not a "sales type" as she put it, as others were. She did not like the politics of the consulting model on which the company was based. As much as I assured her that academic departments were no less brutal, her daily life became a grind. It did not help matters that my daily life in June consisted of the freedom to write from home with a relaxing view of roses and figs right outside my window. While she was being micro-managed, I was doing whatever I wanted.

Coupled with these deep work stresses, and perhaps in some ways related to them, her desire to have a baby was raging again. She was coming towards the time frame that she described as her "last chance to be a mother." I agreed, finally, that we would try—whatever that entailed. I knew that she would be unhappy for a long, long, time, and perhaps resent me, if we did not try as hard as we could to make this work. I also knew that she would be happy if she did have a baby. Her work uncertainty, and the renewed drive to start our own family, brought back some of the same old worries for me. Some of these worries were based on selfishness. If we had a child, would I ever have the enjoyment of retiring? Would we ever create any savings to help us later in life? If she quits her job, and is at home for an extended period of time, how would I get any writing done? How would I save for us while covering her health insurance payments that were now being covered by her workplace? Yet, also, some of the worry was connected to my MacTel. How would we support ourselves if I could no longer work because of blindness? How would Hema support herself, and a baby, if anything happened to me? How useful would I be in raising a child as a blind father? How would Hema cope with a child and a disabled spouse even just in terms of the routines and duties of everyday life—picking them up, dropping them off, and all of the tasks associated with a child's life as they grow up? I left most of these questions unspoken and certainly unanswered. Still she coached me, as ever, to not live in fear, but in my mind these were not just issues of fear, but issues of risk and practicality. What were the best choices for us in guiding our lives together through the unfolding chapters to come, given the uncertainty and unknowns of my health? However, these questions of risk and practicality were awfully difficult for me to separate from those relating to fears and selfishness. They were harder for us to discuss reasonably against a topic as emotionally charged as the last chance to have a baby. Much of this went undiscussed, as we focused on the issues associated with having a child as a woman in her early 40s and a man in my mid 50s.

On the Saturday morning of father's day weekend in mid-June, Hema came to help me pick figs from our garden. The early variety of green figs were just starting to come in, and there were a few ripe fruits on each branch among many that were not yet ready. Many of the branches were now so high that I could not see which clusters had ripe ones among them, especially the ones at the top. To pull every branch down, in turn on both trees, would have been a lot of tiring work for me. So she spotted the ones to pick by their slight change in color—green to pale green, and I hooked the appropriate branches down with a branch trimmer to where we could pick the ripe ones. Sometimes she switched to the task of hooking the branches and pulling them down for me to pick the fruit. The process was not without its tensions as I coached her to twist the figs off gently, and to ease the branches back up into place, so as not to damage the remaining fruit. Soon after, in the kitchen, she cut the first one in half for us to share. It was delicious, bringing on a rare high-five between us. She said something about the high five being more for me as I did most of the work in the garden, and I thought to myself, why would I work so hard at growing things if not for you? The moment passed quickly on into others on a busy day. Yet, somehow, it seemed to me that this small summery scene in and around our garden captured much about our lives together over the past five years.

INDEX

A

B

C

D

E

F

G

H

I

J

K

L

M

N

O

P

R

S

T

U

V

W

Y

Z

Health Communication

Gary L. Kreps, Series Editor

This series examines the powerful influences of human and mediated communication in delivering care and promoting health.

Books analyze the ways that strategic communication humanizes and increases access to quality care as well as examining the use of communication to encourage proactive health promotion. The books describe strategies for addressing major health issues, such as reducing health disparities, minimizing health risks, responding to health crises, encouraging early detection and care, facilitating informed health decisionmaking, promoting coordination within and across health teams, overcoming health literacy challenges, designing responsive health information technologies, and delivering sensitive end-of-life care.

All books in the series are grounded in broad evidence-based scholarship and are vivid, compelling, and accessible to broad audiences of scholars, students, professionals, and laypersons.

For additional information about this series or for the submission of manuscripts, please contact:

Gary L. Kreps
University Distinguished Professor and Chair, Department of Communication
Director, Center for Health and Risk Communication
George Mason University Science & Technology 2, Suite 230, MS 3D6
Fairfax, VA 22030-4444
gkreps@gmu.edu

To order other books in this series, please contact our Customer Service Department:

(800) 770-LANG (within the U.S.)
(212) 647-7706 (outside the U.S.)
(212) 647-7707 FAX

Or browse online by series:
www.peterlang.com

www.ingramcontent.com/pod-product-compliance
Ingram Content Group UK Ltd.
Pitfield, Milton Keynes, MK11 3LW, UK
UKHW021852100926
8556IPUK00020B/1187

9 781433 138300